UNDERSTANDING
EQUINE
MEDICATIONS

REVISED EDITION

UNDERSTANDING
EQUINE
MEDICATIONS
Your guide to horse health care and management

REVISED EDITION

BY BARBARA D. FORNEY, MS, VMD

*the*HORSE *HEALTH CARE LIBRARY*

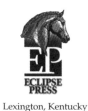

ECLIPSE PRESS

Lexington, Kentucky

Library of Congress Control Number: 2006932558

ISBN-13: 978-1-58150-151-3

ISBN-10: 1-58150-151-X

Printed in the United States

First Edition: 2001

Revised Edition: 2007

Distributed to the trade by

National Book Network

4501 Forbes Blvd., Suite 200

Lanham, MD 20706

1.800.462.6420

Contents

Introduction 6

Chapter 1 8
How To Use This Book

Chapter 2 16
Drug Rules for Competition Horses

Chapter 3 24
Administration of Medication

Chapter 4 32
Medical Math

The Drugs 38
Acepromazine through Xylazine

Appendices 233
Index to Generic and Brand Names 234
References 237
Photo Credits 239
Acknowledgments 239
About the Author 240

Introduction

D rugs and medications are an unavoidable fact of life. People get sick. Animals get sick. Beyond treating infectious disease, veterinarians prescribe drugs for musculoskeletal problems and metabolic diseases, for pain relief, as sedation for other procedures, and for a host of other uses. Horse owners, in particular, are frequently asked to take an active role in treating their horses. In many instances in which one might admit a dog or cat into a veterinary hospital, the horse owner is willing and able to provide nursing care at home. This includes administering both oral and injectable prescription medications. Some horse owners are such terrific nurses that we are able to manage difficult cases at home principally due to their commitment and skill.

Horses are unique among domestic animals because they serve many roles, from the first pony whose main job is to stand still and share carrots or jellybeans with a toddler to the elite world-class athlete that runs faster or jumps higher than most of us can even imagine. I have been fortunate to work with many of these different kinds of horses. The geographic area in which I practice has large breeding operations as well as racehorses, timber horses, three-day-eventing horses, dressage horses, pleasure horses, endurance horses, and almost any other horse you can imagine. These different groups frequently have unique medical needs. Competition horses are under a certain amount of stress due to their training and competition schedule. They need to remain in top athletic form, while their owners/trainers need to be cognizant of, and in compliance with, the drug rules for their sport. There are a number of drugs used in broodmare practice that are not used in any other context. Foals have different medical problems than adult horses, and older horses have unique medical problems associated with aging. Some breeds of horses can have medical problems unique to their breed. Horses can be business investments or lawn ornaments. We love, respect, and have a responsibility toward them whether they are making us money or providing companionship.

A few years ago I was helping some friends write a book for dog and cat owners that covered commonly used medications. It was a little odd that I was involved in this project, as I am an equine practitioner and have been for my whole career. But that project planted the seed that led to this book. As veterinarians we have access to numerous books, articles, and research papers that discuss different drugs, the indications for their use, and their possible side effects. I thought it would be helpful to horse owners and their veterinarians to write a book that discusses some commonly prescribed medications.

This book is by no stretch of the imagination a complete reference guide to all the medications that your veterinarian might prescribe. It is limited to the more common drugs. My intent is to provide an easy-to-use book that is inexpensive enough to leave in your tack trunk, medicine cabinet, or wherever you are most likely to look something up. This book is not in any way intended to be used as a "do it yourself" guide. Its sole purpose is to educate. I hope it will help answer some questions and perhaps generate some questions about the drugs prescribed by your veterinarian.

It is easy and tempting to skip the "HOW TO" section of any book, but take a minute and read this one. There is important general information, as well as safety information, in that section that is not repeated in the individual drug monographs.

Barbara Forney
Coatesville, Pa., 2006

How To Use This Book

The drug monographs in this book are intended only as edu-
cational resources. A concerted effort has been made to provide accurate dosages and up-to-date information. Be aware
that these may change as our knowledge progresses, and errors can
and do occur. If there is a question regarding any information,
including dosages, consult your veterinarian, other references, and
package inserts.

Your veterinarian is the best source of information regarding
diagnosis, treatment, and appropriate drug use and dose. Never
rely on or use information in this book without conferring with
your veterinarian. If the information in this book is not in agree-
ment with your veterinarian's recommendation, discuss it with
your veterinarian, and always follow your veterinarian's instructions. He or she is the one who is examining your horse and has the
best understanding of the medical circumstances. That is why he
or she is your veterinarian.

Drug Monograph Setup

The drugs in this book are listed in alphabetical order by their generic or chemical name. Drugs only have one chemical name, but there
can be many brand names. The index includes both generic names
and some of the common brand names. The drug type and indications

```
┌─────────────────────────────────────────────────┐
│                 AT A GLANCE:                    │
│                 DRUG NAME                       │
│  GENERIC NAME              COMMON BRAND NAME     │
│                                                 │
│  DRUG TYPE                 INDICATIONS          │
│                                                 │
└─────────────────────────────────────────────────┘
```

tell you the general type of drug (such as a tranquilizer or antibiotic) and the medical conditions for which this drug might be used.

Basic Information

This section discusses how the drug works and information about the medical problems for which it might be prescribed.

Side Effects, Precautions, and Overdose

This section covers side effects or known adverse reactions, any special precautions, and information on safety and overdose.

Drug Interactions

This section lists the other drugs whose actions may be affected by this drug. Some drug interactions can be very serious or even fatal.

The horse owner frequently is the only one who is aware of all the medications his or her animal is receiving. You should keep a copy of your horse's medical records so that you may discuss any new medications with your veterinarian. This is particularly true if your horse is seen by more than one veterinarian or is being referred to a hospital.

Special Considerations

This section provides more in-depth information and information that may only be needed under special circumstances. It also discusses some less common uses for the drug and areas of controversy.

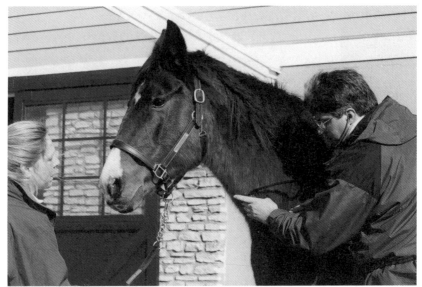

Older horses are among the special populations discussed.

Special Populations

Breeding Animals, Foals, Ponies, Geriatrics, Draft Breeds

This section covers any additional information about the use or safety of the drugs in these special populations. Frequently there is little specific information available about how a drug works in the horse, and your veterinarian may need to extrapolate from information in other species or from his or her own clinical experience.

Competition Horses

This section gives general information regarding the use of this drug in competition horses. Drug-testing methods and drug rules change, and individual horses vary in their clearance of drugs. This information is not intended to provide specific guidance about detection or withdrawal times. Always check with the governing body for your show or competition.

Dose and Route of Administration

Dose range, route of administration, and frequency of administration. How the drug is packaged or provided.

FDA Approval and Off Label or Extra Label Use

The Food and Drug Administration is the federal agency that oversees and controls the licensing, manufacturing, and sale of drugs in the United States. You will see throughout this book the phrase: "U.S. federal law restricts the use of this drug by or on the lawful written or oral order of a licensed veterinarian within the context of a valid veterinarian-client-patient relationship." That simply means it is a prescription drug and should be prescribed by the veterinarian who is treating your horse.

This book also includes information on some drugs that are not FDA approved in the horse. Extra-label use is common in all animal species, not just in horses. FDA approval requires testing to show that the drug is safe and effective at the recommended dose for the indicated diseases in every species for which approval is granted. This type of rigorous testing is very expensive. Frequently, the veterinary market for a given drug is not large enough for the drug companies to justify the cost. As a result, the required safety studies and clinical trials may not have been performed for many drugs commonly used in horses. Much of the information that we have for these drugs is extrapolated from other species, small or informal studies, and clinical use.

Fortunately, veterinarians are able to use a large number of important drugs "extra label" or "off label" provided they are used in a medically responsible fashion within a valid veterinarian-client-patient relationship. There are very specific regulations on extra label drug use, particularly in animals intended for human consumption. The FDA is responsible for animal drug approval, mandates specific withdrawal times for approved drugs, and regulates extra label use. This information and the issue of drug residues are not covered in this book. More information can be found on the FDA Center for Veterinary Medicine Web site at www.fda.gov/cvm.

Proprietary, Generic, and Compounded Drugs

Drugs are categorized into three groups based on how they are manufactured. The first type is the proprietary drugs or "brand name" drugs. These are the new drugs that are still on patent for their manufacturer. They are usually more expensive because the manufacturer needs to recoup the research, development, and testing costs associated with FDA approval.

The second type is the generic drugs. These are drugs that are no longer under patent and are usually sold by their chemical name. As a rule they are cheaper than the original brand name drug. Generic drugs are still regulated under the FDA and must be tested in order to document their "bioequivalence" with the original proprietary drug.

Finally there are compounded drugs. Compounding has become a very large field in veterinary medicine and in some specialties in human medicine. Compounded drugs are made to order at a compounding pharmacy when the proprietary or generic drug is either not available or only available in a formulation that makes it difficult to use. Compounding pharmacies can also make custom mixtures of drugs to treat specific conditions.

Safe Use of Medications

• Store medication in the original container. Be sure the label stays on the container. Throw away any unlabeled containers.

• The medication prescribed by your veterinarian is NOT FOR HUMAN USE.

• Store all medication out of reach of children. Consult your physician immediately if there is any ingestion or other exposure to medication prescribed for your horse.

• Follow your veterinarian's instructions exactly. If you have any questions, contact your veterinarian.

• Dispose of unused or out-of-date medicine in a responsible fashion. Syringes and needles should be disposed of in medical-waste containers. Consult your veterinarian if you have any questions about disposal.

• Do not use medication that is prescribed for one horse on another horse. What is effective and safe for one animal may not be safe or appropriate for another.

• Follow administration directions carefully.

• Be sure to follow any special storage instructions listed on the drug package such as "refrigerate," "do not freeze," or "keep in a cool place." In particular, always avoid extreme hot or cold temperatures.

• Contact your veterinarian immediately if you think your horse is having an adverse reaction to any medication.

• Make sure your veterinarian knows about all of the medications and supplements, including homeopathic and herbal remedies that your horse is taking, and keep records for your own reference.

• If you move or change veterinarians, request that a copy of your horse's medical records be sent to your new veterinarian.

Key to the Monographs

Following are a few terms that appear in a number of the drug monographs:

Aerobic and anaerobic bacteria: Aerobic bacteria require oxygen to live. Anaerobic bacteria only live where there is no oxygen present.

Gram-positive and Gram-negative bacteria: The Gram stain is a staining technique used to help identify different bacteria when they are examined under a microscope. Developed by Danish microbiologist Hans Christian Gram, the Gram stain is simple, quick, and inexpensive, and it is one of the most commonly used stains in microbiology.

Gram-positive bacteria have a relatively simple cell wall, which takes up and retains this stain. Gram-positive bacteria will be stained blue when seen under the microscope. Some examples of Gram-positive bacteria are *Streptococcus* and *Staphylococcus*.

The cell wall of Gram-negative bacteria is multi-layered and more complex. As a result of this difference, these bacteria do not retain the Gram stain. Gram-negative bacteria will appear red when looked at under the microscope. Many of the bacteria normally found in the gastrointestinal tract are Gram-negative. Some examples of are *E. coli*, *Klebsiella*, and *Salmonella*.

Because the cell wall is an important bacterial defense against antibiotics, many antibiotic susceptibility patterns correspond to the

Gram-staining characteristics of the bacteria.

Bactericidal and bacteriostatic antibiotics: Bactericidal antibiotics work by killing the bacteria. Bacteriostatic antibiotics work by preventing growth or reproduction of the bacteria. Some antibiotics may be both bactericidal and bacteriostatic. They may be bacteriostatic at low concentrations and bactericidal at higher concentrations or for particularly susceptible bacterial infections. Usually bacteriostatic antibiotics are not combined with bactericidal antibiotics.

What am I looking for? Following are drugs by category:

Antibiotic
Aminoglycoside antibiotics:
  Gentamicin and Amikacin
Ceftiofur
Chloramphenicol
Enrofloxacin
Macrolide antibiotics:
  Erythromycin, Clarithromycin,
  Azithromycin
Metronidazole
Penicillin
Rifampin
Tetracyclines: Doxycycline
  and Oxytetracycline
Trimethoprim Sulfa

Antihistamine
Cyproheptadine
Hydroxyzine
Pyrilamine and Tripelennamine

Antiprotozoal
Nitazoxanide
Ponazuril
Pyrimethamine/Sulfa combination

Bronchodilator
Albuterol
Clenbuterol

Hormone
Anabolic steroids: Boldenone
  and Stanozolol
Corticosteroids
Deslorelin
Human Chorionic Gonadotropin
Oxytocin
Progesterone, Altrenogest
Prostaglandin

**Nonsteroidal
Anti-inflammatory**
Aspirin
Diclofenac Sodium
Flunixin meglumine
Ketoprofen
Meclofenamic acid
Naproxen
Phenylbutazone

Sedative/Tranquilizer
Acepromazine
Detomidine
Reserpine
Romifidine
Xylazine

Ulcer Medication or GI Upset
Bismuth Subsalicylate
Cimetidine and Ranitidine
DSS
N-Butylscopolammonium Bromide
Omeprazole
Sucralfate

Miscellaneous
Atropine
Butorphanol
DMSO
Domperidone
Furosemide
Griseofulvin
Hyaluronic acid
Isoxsuprine
Methocarbamol
Pergolide
Polysulfated Glycosaminoglycan
Trichlormethiazide and
  Dexamethasone Combination

Drug Rules for Competition Horses

There are many good reasons for using drugs and medications in our horses. Drugs are most often used therapeutically in the treatment of disease. Sometimes drugs are used for the purpose of management, safety, or convenience. Alternatively, drugs can be used in an attempt to change a horse's performance and thereby alter the outcome of a competition. In the belief that competitions should reward the best horse, not the best pharmacologist, the governing bodies of competitive horse sports developed drug rules for competition horses.

Individuals who compete their horses need to comply with the drug rules for their sport. Entry or lower-level competitions frequently do not have formal drug rules, but formal medication rules must be followed in higher levels of competition and in all racing. Compliance with drug rules is monitored by testing for residues in urine or blood samples. Violations may result in penalties, fines, and/or suspensions.

Each regulatory agency has its own drug policies, and the owner of a competition horse and his or her veterinarian need to know the rules applicable to their sport before prescribing or administering any medication.

This section provides an overview of the basic philosophy behind some of the rules. It is not a comprehensive discussion of specific rules (which are constantly being modified), so it is important to read a current copy of the rules for your discipline and work with a veterinarian who is familiar with those rules.

Drug Detection

Compliance with drug rules would be easy if someone could determine exactly how long after administration each drug remains in a horse's system at detectable levels. However, this is not the case. The many variables include the individual horse, the testing method prescribed by the governing body, and the wording of the individual rule.

Even the terminology is confusing. Withdrawal time, withholding time, detection time, and clearance time are all terms used to describe a relationship between the administration of a drug and the status of that drug in the animal's system. Although these terms are often used interchangeably, technically they are slightly different. Withdrawal time is the time needed for most horses given recommended doses to have systemic levels decrease to levels acceptable by a regulatory group. Withholding time is the prescribed time required between the last dose and the start of competition. Detection time is the length of time after administration during which the presence of a drug can be determined by a given test. Clearance time is the actual time it takes for a drug to be excreted or eliminated from the system.

Many factors influence drug metabolism and excretion. Perhaps the major factor is the inherent differences among individual animals. Normal encompasses a range that includes most individuals, but some normal animals always fall outside the normal range. An individual horse might eliminate a drug more slowly than normal and test high even if the recommended withholding times were followed. Factors that influence excretion rate include hydration, amount of body fat, urinary pH, and amount of food in the stomach. Stress, sub-clinical infections, and borderline systemic disease are other things that can affect drug metabolism. The dose of a drug, route of administration, number of doses, brand or formulation of a drug, and other concurrent medications or food supplements are other factors that can influence how long the drug remains at detectable levels.

At the regulatory end, different regulatory groups may use different tests that vary in their sensitivity, and the groups may have different allowable residual drug levels. Because some of the newer drug testing methods can pick up the smallest trace of a drug, some of the regulatory groups are re-examining when a drug is likely to have a pharmacologic effect versus how long trace amounts of the drug can be detected. Drug testing may occur on either blood (plasma) or on urine. Following is a short discussion of some of the regulations and enforcement policies of some of the larger regulatory bodies.

Horse Racing

In states that have horse racing there is usually a racing commission that is in charge of developing and enforcing the rules for that state. The Association of Racing Commissioners International (ARCI) is a national organization that researches and recommends rules and policies associated with racing (www.arci.com). Another organization that is emerging in the racing industry is the Racing Medication and Testing Consortium. The RMTC is working toward establishing a uniform medication policy for use in all U.S. racing jurisdictions.

The racing industry relies heavily on the Uniform Classification Guidelines of Foreign Substances compiled by the ARCI. Drugs on this list are classified from 1 to 5 based on their abuse potential. Class 1 and 2 drugs have the highest potential to affect performance and a low likelihood of therapeutic purpose. Morphine is an example of a Class 1 drug. Class 1 and 2 drug violations have the highest recommended suspension and fine. Class 4 and 5 drugs are therapeutic drugs with a low potential to affect performance. Drugs such as cimetidine or DMSO are Class 5 drugs. A positive test for these drugs has the lowest recommended suspension and fine. Some of the Class 3, 4, and 5 drugs may have permissible detection levels. Antibiotics are generally not classified under the ARCI system because they are therapeutic agents without performance-changing potential (procaine penicillin is an exception due to the procaine; see Penicillin Antibiotics).

The ARCI recommends a "no foreign substance rule," but there is some variation among states particularly regarding furosemide and phenylbutazone levels. It is important to remember that what is legal in one state may not be legal in another state. This is even truer when racing outside the United States. Drug policies and drug testing methods can vary greatly among different countries.

In the case of sanctioned steeplechase racing, National Steeplechase Association rules state: "No horse may participate in any race if it has been administered in any manner any forbidden substance other than furosemide as prescribed herein." The rules go on to discuss thoroughly the regulation of furosemide use. These rules may be viewed on the NSA Web site: www.nationalsteeplechase.com.

The Federation Equestre Internationale (FEI)

The Federation Equestre Internationale is the international governing body for many horse sports including the higher levels of international competition for show jumping, dressage, combined driving, eventing, reining, and endurance. The World Equestrian Games, the equestrian events in the Olympic Games, and many other international competitions are FEI competitions. Some classes at United States Equestrian Federation shows are also under FEI rules. The FEI Veterinary Regulations including the medication rules may be viewed on the organization's Web site: www.horsesport.org.

New veterinary rules are in force as of June 2006. The underlying philosophy of the "level playing field" or no drug should be administered that gives a horse an unfair advantage has not changed. But as drug testing has become more sophisticated, extremely minute quantities of drugs can now be detected. This has led to the possibility of an inadvertent positive from a legitimate use of medication long before the competition. The new rules include a list of some commonly used therapeutic drugs with some guidance regarding detection time. There is also a new provision for elective testing prior to competition to determine if a horse will test positive for a therapeutic drug. It is not clear how long in advance one's veterinarian must request the test.

Another new feature in the 2006 drug regulations is a classification system for forbidden drugs. These drugs are now divided into two groups: Class A and Class B. A positive drug test for a Class A drug is considered a more serious violation than for a Class B drug. Class A drugs include sedatives, stimulants, corticosteroids, nonsteroidal anti-inflammatory drugs, muscle relaxants, and other drugs that clearly could affect performance. Class B drugs are considered less likely to influence performance or have the potential for accidental exposure, such as isoxsuprine.

At this time, FEI competitions are still under a "no foreign substance" or drug-free policy, with a few exceptions. These exceptions include the anti-ulcer medications omeprazole, cimetidine, and ranitidine. These medications may be given without filing special paperwork. Altrenogest may be given to mares in FEI competitions after filling out the appropriate paperwork. There are also substances for which the FEI accepts trace amounts because they could be metabolites of normal nutrients. This includes trace amounts of salicylic acid, theobromine, DMSO, and arsenic. The FEI rules clearly state that herbal products may cause a positive drug test despite claims from the manufacturer, and all responsibility lies with the owner of the horse or the owner's representative.

The FEI rules permit the use of antibiotics, intravenous fluids, and some intranasal oxygen under special circumstances. This is explained further in the rules. Additionally, if a horse is injured or becomes ill during an FEI competition, there are provisions in the veterinary regulations for treatment. The ground jury has the authority to decide on an individual basis if the horse may return to competition after treatment. Except in an emergency, permission to treat must be requested in advance. All the treatment must be reported in writing and there is a treatment form in the veterinary regulations.

The intent of the new FEI veterinary rules is to allow rational use of medication prior to competition in an era when minute quantities of many drugs can be detected long after any pharmacologic effect would be felt by the patient. These rules are new enough that it remains to be seen how they will be applied.

United States Equestrian Federation (USEF)

The USEF has a very proactive stand on drug use in performance horses. The USEF drug rules are printed in the *USEF Rule Book*, Section 401-413, and any questions regarding these rules may be directed to the USEF Drugs and Medication Program office at (800) 633-2472.

The first thing that competitors under USEF rules need to ascertain is if their breed, discipline, or group competes under the no foreign substance provisions or the therapeutic substance rules. The endurance divisions, any FEI class, and USEF selection trials are under no foreign substance while most other divisions are under therapeutic substance rules. Some of the breed divisions may have some additional restrictions. For example, the Arabian division has a more restrictive policy regarding anabolic steroids. USEF drug rules are reviewed regularly and are subject to change.

Therapeutic substance rules permit the use of drugs that have a legitimate therapeutic use and are not likely to affect performance. Forbidden substances are described as follows: "Any product is forbidden if it contains an ingredient that is a stimulant, depressant, tranquilizer, local anesthetic, psychotropic (mood and/or behavior altering) substance, drug which might affect the performance of a horse and/or pony or might interfere with drug testing procedures."

The USEF Web site (www.usef.org) has an excellent article, "Practical Advice Regarding the 2001 USEF Drugs and Medications Rule," and a partial list of drugs that are forbidden. It would be impossible to publish a complete list as there are thousands of drugs, and new drugs are constantly coming on to the market. Guidelines for the use of dexamethasone, methocarbamol, and nonsteroidal anti-inflammatory drugs in accordance with the therapeutic sub-stance rules are covered in this article. Additionally, there is a very interesting discussion of herbal supplements and drug detection times. Following these guidelines or recommendations, while not an absolute guarantee, will certainly minimize the possibility of an acci-dental positive drug test during USEF competition.

Article 411, "Conditions for Therapeutic Administrations of Forbidden Substances," is a provision in the USEF rules describing the circumstances when a forbidden substance may be administered for therapeutic purposes such as the treatment of illness or injury. The rules spell out the parameters of therapeutic use, the proper use of the medication report, the proper procedure for filing the medica-tion report with the steward or technical delegate, and the withdraw-al rules for horses. The procedure may be more complex if the horse is competing in a selection trial (see Section K of Article 411).

American Quarter Horse Association (AQHA)

The AQHA rules were modified in 1999 to "allow the use of some medications under a very stringent set of conditions as defined by the addendum to rule 441 of the *AQHA Official Handbook*." There is also a therapeutic medication fact sheet available on the AQHA Web site (www.aqha.com). The new AQHA rules are similar to the USEF therapeutic substance rules, but they are not exactly the same. It is important to read and understand the new AQHA rules before com-peting in a sanctioned Quarter Horse show. Before this rule change, AQHA sanctioned horse shows operated under a drug-free policy.

United States Pony Clubs Inc. (USPC)

Sections 15 and 16 and Appendix C of the USPC Horse Management Rules cover the use of medication at USPC rallies. These rules are available at the USPC Web site (www.ponyclub.org): "Unless medicine is previously prescribed by a veterinarian, mounts should compete free of medication other than dressings for minor wounds or scrapes." The rules go on to describe how to proceed if your horse needs to be on medication at a rally. The competitor must present an explanatory note which is given to the chief horse management judge and reviewed and verified by the competition veterinarian who then reports to the president of the ground jury. Medication may only be given by the owner of the horse or someone designated by the owner of the horse. So while it is not a "drug free" rule, the use of medication must be communicated and is regulated. Drug testing may occur at Pony Club rallies.

American Driving Society (ADS)

Depending on the level of competition, combined driving competitions may be under FEI rules, USEF rules, or ADS rules. Competitions that are under ADS rules (not FEI or USEF competitions) do not at this time have any regulations concerning drug use. The Web site for viewing the veterinary regulations for the ADS is www.americandrivingsociety.org.

United States Eventing Association (USEA)

At USEA-recognized horse trials all levels are governed by the USEF therapeutic substance rules. This is a change from previous years because now even the lower levels are competing under drug rules. The CCI and CIC competitions are governed by FEI rules.

Administration of Medication

The three most common routes for systemic administration of medication or drugs are intravenously (IV), intramuscularly (IM), and orally (PO). Because different medications are suited to different routes of administration, it is important to follow the directions and use the appropriate route. Medications that are safe and effective by one route may be harmful or even fatal when given by another route.

The chemistry of the individual drug and the physiology of horses dictate the route that a drug is given. For example, oral penicillin is not used in the horse because it is not well absorbed and can adversely affect the normal gut flora. It is well absorbed and works well in dogs, cats, and humans, but not in horses. Imagine how much easier treating an uncomplicated respiratory infection in a foal would be if one could use bubblegum-flavored oral amoxicillin, but, unfortunately, it would not work.

Drugs administered by different routes are also absorbed in different fashions and at different rates. Each route has advantages and disadvantages. The next sections discuss some features of IV, IM, and oral medications.

Intravenous (IV) Medication

Veterinarians give most intravenous injections. Although horses have large jugular veins and the technique for administering IV injections is not very difficult, the patient must stand still and the medication must be accurately placed in the vein rather than around it or in an artery. Drugs that leak or are injected around a vein can be very irritating to the surrounding tissue, causing pain, swelling, and scar tissue formation. The potential complications of IV injection are severe enough that most veterinarians and horse owners feel more

AT A GLANCE: IV

◆ Intravenous medication is injected directly into a vein and the horse's blood stream.

◆ The response to the medication is faster and drug levels peak sooner than with IM injection or oral medication.

◆ The body also metabolizes the drug faster after IV injection, and systemic drug levels decrease sooner than with other forms of administration.

comfortable with veterinary administration. IV injections are usually given in the jugular vein (located on each side of the neck in the "jugular groove"). Sometimes other veins are used in horses whose jugular veins are occluded or infected, but these conditions usually occur after severe or chronic illness requiring multiple intravenous catheters or injections.

Drugs given intravenously are manufactured and stored in a sterile fashion. They need to remain sterile; otherwise bacteria can be injected directly into the bloodstream. The injection site for IV injection should be clean. Swabbing with alcohol is not necessary and is not an effective way to disinfect the area. If the area is very dirty or caked with mud, however, it should be brushed clean or clipped and scrubbed.

The most common serious side effect to intravenous injections is thrombophlebitis, or septic thrombophlebitis. Thrombophlebitis is inflammation due to chemical or mechanical irritation of the wall of the blood vessel. Septic thrombophlebitis means bacterial infection is present in addition to inflammation and irritation. Most minor thrombophlebitis will resolve with appropriate nursing care and nonsteroidal anti-inflammatory drugs, but septic thrombophlebitis is very serious and can be life threatening. Irritation due to thrombophlebitis from intravenous injections of the left jugular vein also can damage the nerve that controls the left side of the larynx. When this occurs, the horse can develop partial paralysis of the arytenoid cartilage of the larynx and become a "roarer." Roarer describes the noise made by horses with partial or complete paralysis of the arytenoid cartilage. The paralyzed cartilage droops, partially occluding the larynx, causing a characteristic noise when the horse exercises. Horses with paralysis of the arytenoid cartilage frequently have some exercise intolerance.

Another serious and dramatic side effect to intravenous injection is intra-arterial injection (into an artery). The carotid artery runs directly behind the jugular vein. It is possible to pass a needle all the way through the jugular vein into the artery and accidentally inject the medication into the carotid artery. Blood in the jugular vein goes to the heart and circulates in the blood throughout the body. Consequently, the injected drug is well mixed and diluted before arriving at the brain. When a drug is accidentally injected in the carotid artery, it goes directly to the brain before having any significant chance for dilution. The brain is hit with a highly concentrated solution of the drug. Intra-carotid injections of drugs can cause collapse, seizures, and death. The onset of signs due to intra-carotid injection are very rapid. The horse may "drop off the needle," a graphic expression that means that the adverse reaction starts as the injection is finished.

When a horse is on long-term intravenous medication or on medication that must be given frequently, such as IV penicillin, many veterinarians will place an intravenous catheter in the jugular vein. The technology associated with large-animal catheters has improved dramatically in the past 10 years. Some wonderful catheters for long-term use that are not irritating to the interior of the blood vessel are available. In some instances the patient/horse can be treated at home even when the medication must be given frequently.

Intramuscular (IM) Medication

Many horse owners are very comfortable giving their horse shots in the muscle. It is not as technically difficult as giving injections into a vein, and there are fewer potentially serious side effects. That is not to say that giving IM injections is risk free.

First, if you want to learn to give IM injections to your horse, plan ahead. Make an appointment with your veterinarian to learn where and how to give a shot. There are pictures in this book and in many others that show where it is safe to give an IM injection, but it may not be as simple as it looks in a

AT A GLANCE: IM

◆ Drugs administered by the IM route are absorbed more slowly than if given IV.

◆ Peak drug levels after IM administration tend to be lower than peak levels after IV administration, but the drug is usually in the system longer.

photo when you are standing there for the first time, needle in hand.

Second, learn the anatomy. IM injections should go deep in the muscles of the neck or in the large muscle of the hindquarters. Some people also use the pectoral muscles of the chest and the gluteal muscles on top of the rump. Each site has its pros and cons. The neck is easy to inject, and you are not likely to be kicked. It is important to inject in the proper area, avoiding the spine on the bottom, the scapula toward the rear, and the nuchal ligament on the top.

There are fewer places for potential error in the large muscles that go down the back of the leg, but the possibility of getting kicked is

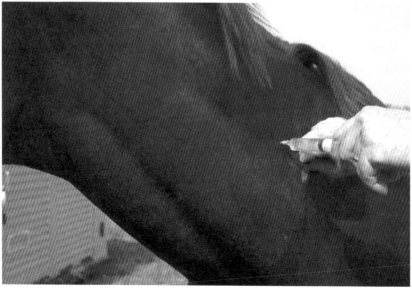

A horse receiving an intramusclar injection in the neck.

much higher. The muscles on the top of the rump are also quite large, but injection site reactions are very difficult to manage at this location due to poor ventral drainage. The pectoral muscles between the front legs are not commonly used. They have the best ventral drainage but are more likely to show swelling.

IM injections must go in the muscle and not in the vein. Many IM drugs are dangerous, or even fatal, if injected IV. Procaine penicillin is probably the best known for causing violent reactions, including convulsions and even death, if accidentally injected into the bloodstream. Proper injection technique is important. Always pull back on the plunger of the syringe once it is placed in the muscle to see if any blood is drawn into the syringe. There are blood vessels throughout all muscles, and it is easy to place a needle right beside a blood vessel or have the end of the needle in a blood vessel. Once it is clear that no blood is aspirated into the syringe, proceed with the injection. No more than 10 to 15 mls of drug should be injected at any one site.

Although uncommon, any injection of medication can cause an allergic or anaphylactic reaction.

Injection site reactions are a common but usually less serious side effect of IM injections. Injection site reactions can vary from minor swelling with heat and tenderness to a deep and serious abscess. Some drugs are more likely to cause an injection site reaction than others, but all drugs have the potential to do so. Some vaccines and drugs are notorious for causing reactions, and some individual horses seem to develop a bump or reaction to almost every shot.

If your horse develops an abscess from an injection, it will usually come to a head, rupture, and drain. Hot compresses are frequently helpful in speeding resolution of an abscess. Drainage is easy and obvious from the neck, hindleg, and pectoral muscles because of the path of gravity. Drainage of an abscess from an injection site reaction in the gluteals is much more of a problem. Some veterinarians may use ultrasound to find and open a fluid pocket in a difficult abscess.

Horses with an injection site reaction in the neck will hold their heads and necks at a stiff and peculiar angle. They may be unwilling to move their head and neck and may need to have their hay and water raised to a level at which they can eat and drink comfortably. Injection site reactions in the leg or hip usually present as stiffness or lameness. There are rarely any long-term serious consequences to injection site reactions, and most of them resolve

AT A GLANCE: PO
◆Oral administration is the slowest route for absorption.
◆The oral route of administration is the least likely to cause adverse reactions.
◆Blood levels from oral medication usually approach those of intramuscular medication.

with good nursing care although occasionally the more serious ones can take months to heal.

Injections hurt, and that includes IM injections. Some horses are easy to give shots to, but some horses become dangerous when faced with a needle and a syringe. There are many ways to manage the injection-shy or fearful horse, but get advice or help before anyone gets hurt.

Drugs for intramuscular injection are manufactured and stored in sterile bottles. Injection sites should be clean. Do not reuse needles. Make sure drugs are stored properly to minimize the possibility of contamination with bacteria. Always follow your veterinarian's directions or those on the package insert concerning proper drug storage. Discuss with your veterinarian the appropriate disposal of any unused medicine, syringes, and needles. They are considered hazardous medical waste.

Oral (PO) Medication

Administering oral medication is simple and painless. All of us, our horses included, would probably rather receive our medication in an oral form. The use of oral medication does not require any sterile equipment, causes few adverse effects, and is particularly handy for long-term treatment. The only real disadvantage is that some animals are difficult to dose, and the only way any medication is going to work is if it gets into the horse's system. It does not work if most of it ends up on the ground. The abbreviation that is commonly used for oral dosing is PO, which stands for "per os" or "by mouth."

Oral medication in powder form may be dosed by sprinkling on a grain ration or by dissolving in a sweet liquid such as molasses and giving by dose syringe. Many horses are suspicious of medication in their grain and may not eat. If you are attempting to medicate in the grain, make sure that the grain is eaten and that the medication is not sifted out and left behind. Sometimes the addition of molasses or other sticky sweetener helps bind the powder to the kernels of grain.

Pills may be dissolved and squirted in the horse's mouth, ground up and top dressed as a powder on grain, or placed in the back of the mouth using an apparatus called a balling gun. The balling-gun approach is used much less frequently these days. It takes practice to be proficient and many horses resent having a long instrument placed firmly in the back of their mouths. Dissolving the pills in hot water flavored with any of a variety of sweeteners is a common approach. Disposable catheter tip syringes (60 ml) are an easy, inexpensive piece of equipment that can be used repeatedly. Most veterinarians stock them or can order them. The syringe will last much longer if it is taken apart and rinsed after use. Some people also use turkey basters or the large volume livestock dose syringes, depending on the medication volume and their personal preference. A wide range

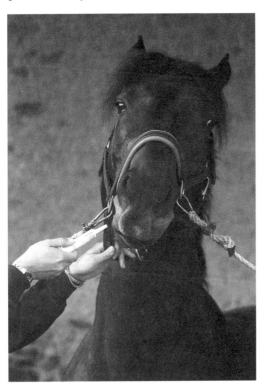

A horse receiving oral medication.

of products may be used as sweetener, including molasses, honey, pancake syrup, gelatin, soft drink mix, frozen apple juice concentrate, and applesauce. It helps to experiment and work out how to dose an individual with the least struggle, particularly when working with a horse that is on long-term medication. Veterinary compounding pharmacies can specially mix drugs in a variety of concentrations and flavors.

Paste formulations of medication are very common. To a great extent, the taste of the paste and the horse's previous experience with oral medication will influence technique. Paste formulations have enough "body" that the experienced "wise-guys" can spit them right back at you if they are so inclined. Placing the paste far back on the tongue and elevating the head after squirting in the medication can help keep most of the paste in the horse. Some paste formulations become runnier when held under warm water. Depending on the horse, a runny formulation may be swallowed more easily. The best techniques combine keeping the paste in the patient with minimal struggle or discomfort to everyone.

4

Medical Math

We all have had that unsure moment where we stood looking at the bottle and then the syringe and then at the directions. Something just did not seem quite right. Did I hear correctly? Or maybe I wrote down the information incorrectly. This section will give you the tools to confirm your veterinarian's prescription and dose. In the final analysis, if things do not add up and make sense, call your veterinarian. It is much better to double check directions than to make a mistake that could endanger your horse.

Calculating dose is the same basic mathematical problem, no matter in what form the drug is supplied.

$$\frac{\text{Dose Rate X Weight of your horse}}{\text{Concentration of Drug}} = \text{Amount of drug to give}$$

Calculating Doses

Dose Rate

First you need to know the recommended dose rate. Dose rate is also frequently called dose, as in "what dose do I give?" In that context, the answer to that question can be confusing. It could be given either as the amount of drug per pound or the total amount of drug to be given to the animal. I used the term dose rate in this explanation to differentiate from the total dose of the drug to be given. Dose rate is how much of the drug to give per pound or per kilogram of body weight. This is usually expressed as the number of mg/lb (milligrams per pound) or mg/kg (milligrams per kilogram). This book gives dose rates in mg/lb. Most veterinary texts express them in mg/kg. We all supposedly "went metric" about 20 years ago, but some of us have not quite gotten there yet and still think of horses in terms of pounds. There are 2.2 lbs in a kg. If a dose rate is expressed in mg/kg and you are more comfortable working in pounds, you should divide the dose by 2.2 to convert to mg/lb.

AT A GLANCE

◆ All medication should be prescribed by your veterinarian, who also should determine and calculate all doses.

◆ If the dose range in this book does not agree with the dose prescribed by your veterinarian, follow your veterinarian's recommendation.

◆ This information is provided to give the reader the tools to understand how doses are derived.

So for example:

If the dose rate is 12 mg/kg, divide by 2.2 = 5.5 mg/lb.

If the dose rate is 100 mg/kg, divide by 2.2 = 45 mg/lb.

Weight

Second, you need to know how much your horse or pony weighs. Most veterinarians are reasonably good at estimating weight. We do it all day long and occasionally get to confirm our estimates using a large animal scale.

Weight tapes are very useful in estimating weight. They are reasonably accurate for most breeds and cheap. If you have the opportunity to weigh your horse on a scale, you can double-check the accuracy of the weight tape for your horse.

Drug Concentration

Third, you need to know how the medication is supplied or know its concentration.

Drugs are usually manufactured as liquids, tablets, capsules, boluses (large soft tablets), powder for reconstitution, powder for top dressing, or paste.

The concentration of most liquid medications is expressed as mg/ml (milligrams per milliliter) and is always stated on the label. It is important to remember that some drugs are sold in several different concentrations, and it is essential to read the label every time.

Tablets and boluses consist of an inactive powder and a drug that are compressed. Capsules are usually made of gelatin and contain the drug and inactive powder. The inactive ingredients make it easier to manufacture the pills in standard sizes. Pills and capsules have the number of milligrams/tablet listed on the label. Some pills are scored and can be split. Pills that are not scored sometimes do not have the drug evenly distributed within the pill and should not be split. Again, pills and capsules can come in different strengths, and it is essential to read the label every time.

Some drugs such as penicillin G and ceftiofur are supplied as a sterile powder to be reconstituted with water or saline to make a liquid. The final concentration depends on how many milliliters of liquid are added to the bottle. Your veterinarian will decide what concentration is appropriate. Usually on the label or package insert there are directions that say how much liquid must be added to get the required concentration. Once the product is diluted, the dose is calculated in the same way as it is for other liquid preparations. Products that need reconstitution frequently have a limited shelf life once they are prepared, and some require refrigeration. Read and follow the package directions about how to store the drug and how long it may be used after reconstitution.

Powders usually have the number of milligrams/packet of powder marked on the label. The powder is sprinkled on top of or mixed with the feed.

Most paste products come in syringes with the amount of products or dose rate marked on the plunger. The proper dose is administered by moving a ring on the plunger to the desired mark and depressing the plunger. The ring can be locked in place to prevent the plunger from pushing out more than the required dose. Lock the ring in position to prevent accidental overdose.

Applying the Equation

As we said at the beginning of this section, calculating dose is always the same basic mathematical problem. You may be worried about miscalculating the number of zeros or the decimal place particularly since you may be converting from milligrams to grams when multiplying out the amount of drug to give. With practice and a calculator, this exercise will become less of a mystery; especially since we are confirming the dose given by your veterinarian, so the answer is already known.

$$\frac{\text{Dose Rate (mg/lb) X Weight (lbs)}}{\text{Concentration (mg/ml or mg/pill)}} = \text{Amount of drug to give}$$

When working with a liquid:

1) Multiply the dose rate (in mg/lb) times your horse's weight (in lbs). Remember to be consistent in either kilograms or pounds. That will give you the total number of milligrams for the dose for your horse.

2) Next divide that number by the concentration of the drug (in mg/ml). That will give you the number of milliliters (ml) of drug to give.

Sample problem for liquids:

Dose Rate = 10 mg/lb; Weight = 1,200 lbs
Concentration of liquid = 500 mg/ml

$$\frac{10 \text{ mg/lb X 1,200 lbs}}{500 \text{ mg/ml}} = \frac{12,000 \text{ mg}}{500 \text{ mg/ml}} = 24 \text{ ml}$$

When working with tablets, pills, or capsules:

1) Multiply the dose rate (mg/lb) times your horse's weight (in lbs). Remember to be consistent in either kilograms or pounds.

2) Divide by the number of milligrams in the pill or capsule. That will give you the number of pills to give.

Sample problem for pill or capsule:

Dose Rate =20 mg/lb; Weight = 600 lbs
Concentration in capsule = 300 mg/capsule

$$\frac{20 \text{ mg/lb X 600 lbs}}{300 \text{ mg/capsule}} = \frac{1,200 \text{ mg}}{300 \text{ mg}} = 4 \text{ capsules}$$

Dose Schedule

Pharmacokinetics is the study of how a drug is absorbed and metabolized by the body. This determines how much and how often a drug is given. The pharmacokinetics for many drugs can vary among species. It is very important to follow directions precisely both in terms of amount and frequency of administration. When a drug is prescribed for three times a day, that means once every eight hours, not three times when it is convenient. A sample schedule for three-times-a-day dosing would be 8 a.m., 4 p.m., and 12 midnight. Likewise, twice-a-day dosing could be 6 a.m. and 6 p.m., not a lopsided day such as 8 a.m. and 4 p.m.

Handy Units of Measure

Weight

Kilograms: kg: 1,000 grams.

Grams: g: 1/1,000 of a kg.

Milligrams: mg: 1/1,000 of a g.

Micrograms: ug: 1/1,000 of a mg.

Pounds: lb: 0.45 kg or 2.2 lbs in a kg.

International Unit: IU.

Grain: 64.8 mg.

Volume

Liter: L: 1,000 ml.

Milliliter: ml: 1/1,000 Liter.

Cubic Centimeter: cc: is the volume of 1 ml of water. When measuring liquid medicine, cc and ml are interchangeable. For example, if the dose is 5 ml and the syringe is marked in cc, give 5 cc.

Teaspoon: tsp: 5 ml.

Tablespoon: tbs: 3 tsp or 15 ml.

Ounce: oz: 30 mls or 2 tbs.

Quart: qt: 0.95 Liter.

AT A GLANCE:

ACEPROMAZINE

GENERIC NAME
Acepromazine maleate

Promazine hydrochloride

COMMON BRAND NAME
Aceproject,
PromAce Injectable
Promazine Granules

DRUG TYPE
Phenothiazine tranquilizer

INDICATIONS
Tranquilization, sedation

Basic Information

Acepromazine maleate is a phenothiazine tranquilizer. Information in this profile also applies to promazine hydrochloride, a similar, milder tranquilizer.

Acepromazine is one of the most commonly used tranquilizers for horses. It decreases anxiety and causes central nervous system depression. It also causes a drop in blood pressure. It is usually given by injection in the muscle (IM) or in the vein (IV) although it also may be given orally. Acepromazine does not relieve pain, and its tranquilizing effect can be overcome unexpectedly, particularly by sensory stimulation such as loud noise or increased activity in the area. It may be less effective if given after the horse is excited. There is a great deal of individual variability in the response to acepromazine, and some horses need much lower doses than others.

Because acepromazine lowers blood pressure by dilating small blood vessels, it is sometimes prescribed for laminitis in an effort to improve circulation in the hoof. Acepromazine may be used in horses that are prone to tie up, both as a preventative measure or as a part of the treatment. When acepromazine is used to treat a tied-up horse, intravenous fluids also may be used to increase hydration and support kidney function.

Side Effects, Precautions, and Overdose

• Acepromazine lowers blood pressure: it should not be used in animals that are dehydrated, anemic, or in shock.

• Because acepromazine lowers blood pressure, it is generally not used in horses with colic.

• Penile paralysis can occur in male horses.

• Acepromazine lowers the hematocrit or packed cell volume (PCV) by 25% to 50%. This effect occurs within 30 minutes of administration and may last for 12 hours or more. This may result in a misdiagnosis of anemia if blood samples are taken after acepromazine administration.

• With any form of sedation, horses can react suddenly and unexpectedly. Always work carefully around a sedated horse no matter how "asleep" it may appear.

• Overdose will cause excessive sedation, slow breathing and heart rate, pale gums, unsteady gait, poor coordination, and inability to stand.

Drug Interactions

• Animals receiving acepromazine will require lower doses of barbiturates, narcotics, and other anesthetics because these combinations will increase central nervous system depression.

• Acepromazine should not be used in horses recently wormed with a piperazine compound.

Special Considerations

• When sedating a horse using acepromazine, it is important to wait until the drug has taken effect before beginning any procedure. Intravenous acepromazine will take about 15 minutes; intramuscular acepromazine will not take full effect for about 30 to 45 minutes.

• The effects of acepromazine will last from one to four hours, but this varies significantly among individual horses. Some very sensitive horses appear slightly sedated for up to 24 hours.

• Some veterinarians use acepromazine in the post-foaling mare with a suspected uterine artery rupture to keep her quiet and decrease further bleeding by lowering blood pressure. A ruptured uterine artery is a life-threatening emergency, and the best treatment is still controversial. Some veterinarians lower the mare's blood pressure with drugs such as acepromazine while others take the opposite approach by supporting the mare's blood pressure with high volumes of intravenous fluids, including hypertonic saline. Both of these contradictory approaches have their supporters.

• Acepromazine is FDA approved for use in horses and requires a prescription. U.S. federal law restricts this drug to use by or on the lawful written or oral order of a licensed veterinarian within the context of a valid veterinarian-client-patient relationship.

Special Populations

Breeding Animals

Most reference books state that acepromazine and other sedatives should be avoided in pregnancy or lactation unless the benefits of using the drug outweigh the risks. Some veterinarians use low doses of acepromazine in apprehensive maiden mares after foaling to persuade the mare to allow the foal to nurse. Although acepromazine has been shown to be excreted in the milk, at low doses this is rarely a problem. Penile paralysis is a rare but recognized side effect to acepromazine. This drug should only be used in breeding stallions after careful consideration of the risk.

Foals

Acepromazine can affect an animal's ability to regulate its temperature. It should be avoided or used with caution in very young foals. Because acepromazine lowers blood pressure, it is generally not used in sick foals.

Ponies

Pony breeds do not appear to differ from horses in their response to acepromazine.

Geriatrics

Acepromazine should be used with caution in older animals because of the lowering of blood pressure. If used, a lower dose should be considered.

Draft Horses

Draft horse breeds are especially sensitive to most sedatives. When acepromazine is used in draft horse breeds, it is generally used at a lower dose.

Competition Horses

Acepromazine is a prohibited substance in most sanctioned competitions. USEF has provisions in its rules for the therapeutic use of prohibited substances. Acepromazine is also a prohibited class A medication under the new FEI rules. It may be detected in the blood for approximately 72 to 120 hours, depending on the number of doses and the sensitivity of the test. Long-term or repeated doses can cause positive tests for weeks or months. Oral use of acepromazine can also increase the detection time.

Dose and Route of Administration

Oral: Promazine HCL: 0.5 to 1.0 mg/lb

Injectable: Acepromazine: 0.01 to 0.03 mg/lb, IV or IM

Dose Form: Injectable 10 mg/ml

Granules containing 27.5 mg of promazine/gram

AT A GLANCE:
ALBUTEROL

GENERIC NAME
Albuterol

COMMON BRAND NAME
Proventil, Ventolin

DRUG TYPE
Bronchodilator

INDICATIONS
Bronchospasm, chronic obstructive pulmonary disease, respiratory distress

Basic Information

Albuterol is used in horses to relax smooth muscle surrounding the airways in the lung and open those airways. It is sometimes used in the treatment of chronic obstructive pulmonary disease (COPD) or "heaves." Albuterol may also be used in horses or foals in respiratory distress. Newer bronchodilators such as clenbuterol are more commonly used systemically for the long-term management of COPD and allergic airway disease. Albuterol is well absorbed orally or inhaled as a fine mist (inhaler or nebulizer system). It is not generally recommended orally due to side effects at therapeutic dose levels.

COPD is an inflammatory disease of the lungs in horses, causing the small airways to constrict and become clogged with mucus. COPD is a progressive disease, meaning that horses with COPD are managed, not cured. It is best treated through a combination of husbandry changes and medication. Bronchodilators and corticosteroids are two of the mainstay medications used in the management and treatment of COPD. Husbandry changes include reducing exposure to the dust in hay and barns and to high ammonia concentrations from urine in poorly ventilated stalls.

Inhaled bronchodilators such as albuterol are sometimes used as performance-enhancing drugs, especially in racehorses. The thought behind this use is that bronchodilation will increase oxygen uptake by the blood and increase the amount of oxygen that reaches the muscles. This is not a legal use in most competitions.

Side Effects, Precautions, and Overdose

• Side effects include increased heart rate, trembling, excitement, sweating, colic, and slowing of the gastrointestinal tract. Side effects are generally dose related.

• Inhalation therapy allows a much lower dose, specifically targeting the lungs and airways. This reduces the risk of side effects as compared to oral administration.

• Overdose increases the risk and severity of the above-mentioned side effects.

Drug Interactions

• Albuterol used in combination with other drugs that have a similar mechanism of action increases the risk of cardiovascular side effects.

Special Considerations

• Inhaled albuterol takes effect very rapidly, usually within five minutes; effects last about one hour.

• There has been a lot of progress in metered dose inhaler systems for horses. When planning inhalation therapy, you should remember that the type of inhaler system has a large impact on the dose and treatment schedule. Metered dose inhaler systems are more efficient than many of the nebulizer systems.

• Since clenbuterol was approved and became legal to use in the United States, it has largely replaced albuterol for oral or systemic use.

• Albuterol is not FDA approved in horses, but it is used and considered accepted practice. Albuterol is a prescription drug. U.S. federal law restricts this drug to use by or on the lawful written or oral order of a licensed veterinarian within the context of a valid veterinarian-client-patient relationship.

Special Populations

Breeding Animals

Albuterol crosses the placenta and in large doses causes birth defects in laboratory animals. It is not known if it is excreted in milk. Administration using an inhaler system uses a lower dose and reduces the amount of drug absorbed systemically. This may reduce the risk of side effects in breeding animals. Albuterol should only be used in pregnant mares when the benefits outweigh the potential risks.

Foals

Inhaled albuterol is sometimes used in very sick foals in respiratory distress. It is usually given with supplemental oxygen.

Ponies

Pony breeds do not appear to differ from horses in their response to albuterol.

Geriatrics

Inhaled albuterol is relatively safe in older animals that do not have other medical conditions that increase the risk of using this drug.

Competition Horses

Albuterol is prohibited or regulated in most sanctioned competitions. It is a prohibited class A medication under the new FEI rules. A single oral dose may be detected in urine for 24 to 30 hours. Detection time after inhaled doses may be shorter. Detection may be affected by the number of doses and the sensitivity of the test. There is ongoing research into creating more sensitive methods for detecting inhaled bronchodilators. Some state racing commissions have a threshold detection level.

Dose and Route of Administration

Inhaled: 0.5 to 1.0 micrograms (ug)/lb. As noted earlier, dosing for different inhalation systems will vary. High doses by inhalation (3.0 ug/lb) may cause side effects.

Dose Form: metered dose inhalers, and solution for nebulization, 0.5% and 0.083%

AT A GLANCE:

AMINOGLYCOSIDES

GENERIC NAME	COMMON BRAND NAME
Gentamicin	Gentocin, Gentaject, Gentaved
Amikacin	Amiglyde

DRUG TYPE	INDICATIONS
Antibiotic	Susceptible bacterial infections

Basic Information

There are many aminoglycosides, including gentamicin, amikacin, streptomycin, neomycin, kanamycin, and tobramycin. Gentamicin and amikacin are the most commonly used aminoglycosides in the horse. This is an important group of antibiotics because of their ability to kill Gram-negative bacteria. These antibiotics are not effective against most Gram-positive or anaerobic bacteria. For this reason, they are frequently combined with other antibiotics, such as one of the penicillins, to give more broad-spectrum antibiotic coverage. The aminoglycoside antibiotics are usually reserved for serious illnesses because of the risk of kidney and inner ear toxicity.

Aminoglycosides are poorly absorbed from the gastrointestinal (GI) tract after oral dosing and must be given by injection in the muscle (IM), or in the vein (IV). Some animoglycoside preparations are used topically for skin and eye infections.

The aminoglycosides have been in use since the 1950s, and some bacteria have become resistant, particularly to older members of the group. Amikacin has a broader spectrum than some of the other members of this group and is effective against many of the aminoglycoside-resistant strains of bacteria. It is often used for bacterial infections resistant to gentamicin.

Side Effects, Precautions, and Overdose

• All of the aminoglycoside antibiotics can cause damage to the kidneys and to the inner ear. Horses at the greatest risk for these side effects are young and old animals; horses that are septic, dehydrated, or have a high fever; and those that already have kidney disease.

• Aminoglycosides should not be used in horses with neuromuscular diseases or botulism.

• Injection site reactions such as pain and swelling may occur after intramuscular injection.

• Precautions such as adjusting the dose, maintaining hydration, monitoring blood levels of antibiotic, and monitoring kidney function help to decrease the risk of side effects.

• Overdose causes an increased risk of serious side effects.

Drug Interactions

• Diuretics, such as furosemide, increase the chances of kidney damage from aminoglycosides.

• Aminoglycosides should be avoided or used with caution with other drugs that have potential toxicity to the ear, kidneys, or nervous system.

• Aminoglycosides can increase the effects of some of the drugs used during general anesthesia. It is important to keep accurate records and notify the surgeon of all medications given prior to referral for surgery.

Special Considerations

• Some veterinarians use a once-a-day high dose of gentamicin rather than smaller doses three to four times a day. Some studies suggest that this may reduce the possibility of kidney damage without decreasing the effectiveness.

• The metabolism of animoglycosides can vary a great deal among individuals. This can affect the dose and frequency of administration.

• Gentamicin is approved only for intrauterine use in the horse, but it has been used systemically for years, and is accepted and common practice. Amikacin is not approved for use in the horse, but it is commonly used and accepted practice. U.S. federal law restricts these drugs to use by or on the lawful written or oral order of a licensed veterinarian within the context of a valid veterinarian-client-patient relationship.

Special Populations

Breeding Animals

Results of studies done in other species show that aminoglycosides have not hurt the fetus. However, there have been reports of infants born with hearing loss after their mothers were treated with these drugs during pregnancy. No information is found on secretion into milk or on adverse effects on fertility of stallions.

Foals

Aminoglycosides should be used with extreme caution in very young foals because they are more susceptible to adverse effects. Dose reduction, longer intervals between doses, and monitoring of drug concentration and kidney function are frequently recommended.

Ponies

Pony breeds do not appear to differ from horses in their response to aminoglycoside antibiotics.

Geriatrics

Aminoglycosides should be used with extreme caution in older horses and in horses with kidney problems. Dose reductions, increased dose intervals, and monitoring of drug concentration and kidney function are frequently recommended.

Competition Horses

Aminoglycoside antibiotics are forbidden in drug-free competitions, but many regulatory groups do not prohibit antibiotics. USEF has provisions in its rules for the therapeutic use of prohibited substances; aminoglycoside antibiotics are not restricted under these rules. It is important to check with the individual regulatory organization.

Dose and Route of Administration

Injectable:

Amikacin: 2 to 3 mg/lb, IV or IM, two to three times a day

Or 7 to 9 mg/lb, once a day

Gentamicin: 0.5 to 1.0 mg/lb, IV or IM, two to four times a

day. Or 3 to 4 mg/lb, once a day

Dose Form:

Amikacin: 50 mg/ml

Gentamicin: 50 mg/ml and 100 mg/ml

AT A GLANCE:
ANABOLIC STEROIDS

GENERIC NAME	COMMON BRAND NAME
Boldenone	Equipoise
Stanozolol	Winstrol

DRUG TYPE	INDICATIONS
Anabolic steroid hormone	Appetite stimulation, increased muscle mass, increased bone density, increased red blood cells

Basic Information

Anabolic steroids, such as stanozolol and boldenone, are synthetic derivatives of the male hormone testosterone. They are labeled for use in debilitated or weakened animals to stimulate appetite and increase weight gain, strength, and vigor. Frequently, they are used in racehorses and performance horses to improve strength and try to improve athletic performance. There has been no scientific evidence to show that they actually improve performance such as make a horse run faster. But some trainers think that anabolic steroids will make a horse feel better and train better. Anabolic steroids are a double-edged sword. They are powerful, long-lasting drugs, with the potential for serious side effects.

Side Effects, Precautions, and Overdose

• Side effects of anabolic steroids depend on the dose, choice of drug, and duration of treatment.

• The most common side effects are difficult to control or aggressive behavior, masculine behavior and appearance, and impairment of fertility. Fillies and mares treated with anabolic steroids may show masculine behavior, temporarily stop reproductive cycling, and have hard, small, inactive ovaries. It can be months before they return to normal reproductive function. Males treated with anabolic steroids may have decreased testicular size, decreased sperm numbers, and other adverse effects on reproductive performance.

• Work in other species suggests that anabolic steroids should be used with caution in animals with heart, liver, or kidney problems.

• For intramuscular injection (IM) only.

• No specific information on overdose was found.

Drug Interactions

• Anabolic steroids may increase the effects of warfarin and other anticoagulants.

Special Considerations

• When anabolic steroids are used as they are intended, for short periods of time on patients that are recovering from illness or trauma, the side effects are not as pronounced, or long lasting.

• The effects of anabolic steroids usually last for several weeks.

• Stanozolol and boldenone are FDA approved for use in horses. They are prescription drugs and controlled substances under the Anabolic Steroid Control Act (Schedule III). U.S. federal law restricts the use of this drug by or on the lawful written or oral order of a licensed veterinarian. These drugs are controlled due to the abuse potential by human athletes seeking to increase muscle mass and strength.

Special Populations

Breeding Animals

Anabolic steroids should not be used in pregnant animals due to masculinization of the fetuses. It is not known if anabolic steroids are excreted in milk.

Anabolic steroids should not be used in breeding stallions because of adverse effects on testicular size and sperm production.

Foals

Anabolic steroids should not be used in young animals because they can cause premature closure of growth plates and abnormal sexual development.

Ponies

Pony breeds do not appear to differ from horses in their response to anabolic steroids.

Geriatrics

Anabolic steroids should be safe to use in older horses if liver and kidney functions are adequate.

Competition Horses

Anabolic steroids are prohibited in any drug-free competition. There are very good drug tests for anabolic steroids, which can be detected for months after a single use. If a regulatory group decides to test for them, they will be detected. Different horse racing commissions and regulatory agencies approach anabolic steroids differently although there is some discussion within racing of moving them from a Class 4 drug to a Class 3 drug. Even within the different breed competitions of the USEF, the regulations can vary. It is important to check the rules with each specific group. Anabolic steroids are much more closely regulated outside of North America.

Dose and Route of Administration

Injectable:

Stanozolol: 0.25mg/lb, IM, once every two weeks weekly for up to four injections

Boldenone: 0.5 mg/lb, IM, once every three weeks

Dose Form:

Stanozolol: 50 mg/ml, injectable

Boldenone: 25 mg/ml, injectable

AT A GLANCE:

ANTIHISTAMINES

GENERIC NAME
Pyrilamine maleate
Tripelennamine

COMMON BRAND NAME
Pyrilaject
Re-Covr

DRUG TYPE
Antihistamine

INDICATIONS
Hives, bee stings, itchy
skin, and other allergic
skin problems

Basic Information

Pyrilamine maleate and tripelennamine are antihistamines. They are used to treat allergic problems in horses, such as hives and itchy or bumpy allergic skin reactions. Because pyrilamine maleate and tripelennamine are injectable, they can also be used for allergic reactions such as tongue or facial swelling due to bee sting, insect bite, or contact with an irritating plant.

Histamine is a substance that is released from some types of cells if those cells are damaged. It causes contraction of smooth muscle cells, including those in the respiratory tract and intestines. It lowers blood pressure by causing dilation of blood vessels. It causes the inflammation and itching typical of allergic reactions.

Antihistamines do not block the release of histamine. Instead, they compete with histamine for uptake at the histamine receptors on sensitive cells in the respiratory tract, intestines, blood vessels, and the skin. Oral antihistamines generally take 20 to 45 minutes to take effect. Injectable antihistamines such as pyrilamine maleate and tripelennamine act more rapidly, but they are more likely to cause side effects and are not as commonly used as some of the oral products. If antihistamines alone are unable to control all of the allergic signs, they may be used with corticosteroids, allowing use of a lower dose of the corticosteroids.

Side Effects, Precautions, and Overdose

• Sedation is a common side effect with antihistamine use. Less common side effects include excitement, fine tremors, whole body tremors, and seizures. Gastrointestinal side effects such as colic or loss of appetite are possible.

• Antihistamines may thicken mucus in the respiratory tract. Extra caution should be used in horses with respiratory problems due to excess mucus.

• Pyrilamine should be given slowly intravenously (IV). Rapid administration increases the possibility of side effects.

• Tripelennamine should only be given intramuscularly (IM).

• Individuals may react differently to antihistamines. The dose of pyrilamine or tripelennamine may need to be tailored to the individual horse.

• Overdoses would be expected to cause increased sedation and severity of other side effects.

Drug Interactions

• Antihistamines have an additive effect when combined with other central nervous system depressant drugs, such as tranquilizers.

• Antihistamines may affect the activity of anticoagulants like warfarin.

Special Considerations

• Pyrilamine and tripelennamine are FDA approved for use in horses, and they are prescription drugs. U.S. federal law restricts this drug to use by or on the lawful written or oral order of a licensed veterinarian within the context of a valid veterinarian-client-patient relationship.

Special Populations

Breeding Animals

High doses of antihistamines have been shown to cause birth defects in laboratory animals. It is not known if these drugs are excreted in milk. They should only be used in pregnant or lactating animals if the benefits outweigh the risks.

Foals

If antihistamines are used in a foal, they should be used at a reduced dose.

Ponies

Pony breeds do not appear to differ from horses in their response to antihistamines.

Geriatrics

There are no studies in horses, but older humans are more sensitive to side effects from antihistamines. When using antihistamines in older horses, it may be reasonable to start with a low dose.

Competition Horses

Pyrilamine maleate and tripelennamine are prohibited or regulated in most sanctioned competitions. Pyrilamine maleate may be detected for at least 36 hours in blood or urine after a single dose. Tripelennamine may be detected for 36 to 72 hours. Detection time may vary with the sensitivity of the drug test. Repeated doses may also affect detection times. USEF has provisions in its rules for the therapeutic use of prohibited substances. It is important to consult the individual regulatory group.

Dose and Route of Administration

Injectable:
    Pyrilamine maleate: 0.4 to 0.6 mg/lb, by slow IV injection
    Tripelennamine: 0.5 mg/lb, by deep IM injection
Dose Form:
    Pyrilamine maleate injection: 20 mg/ml
    Tripelennamine hydrochloride: 20 mg/ml

AT A GLANCE:
ASPIRIN

GENERIC NAME
Aspirin
Acetylsalicylic acid

COMMON BRAND NAME
Generics

DRUG TYPE
Nonsteroidal anti-inflammatory
drug (NSAID)

INDICATIONS
Pain relief, fever reduction,
prevention of blood clots,
anti-inflammatory

Basic Information

Aspirin is a nonsteroidal anti-inflammatory drug (NSAID). It is used as a mild pain reliever, fever reducer, and anti-inflammatory. One of its major uses in horses is in the treatment of blood-clotting problems.

NSAIDs work by inhibiting the body's production of prostaglandins and other chemicals that stimulate the body's inflammatory response. Some of their actions may be dose dependent. NSAIDs are quickly absorbed into the blood stream; pain relief and fever reduction usually start within one to two hours.

Aspirin has a very short, effective duration for pain relief but a much longer effect on clotting function. Aspirin slows or prevents platelets from aggregating and sticking to the inside of blood vessels and, therefore, slowing or preventing the formation of blood clots. Aspirin's effect on blood clotting lasts from eight to 10 days.

Aspirin may be used in laminitis, chronic lymphangitis, inflamed or infected veins, and any other disease where blood clot formation contributes to the problem and is, therefore, undesirable. Aspirin is sometimes used for minor lameness problems, but the duration of pain relief is short. Other NSAIDs are more effective. Aspirin is also used as an anti-inflammatory for some eye problems.

Side Effects, Precautions, and Overdose

• The most common side effect is gastrointestinal (GI) irritation and bleeding.

• When aspirin is used frequently at higher doses, such as for musculoskeletal problems, other typical NSAID side effects include kidney damage, bleeding disorders, and protein loss.

• Rare allergies to aspirin may occur. The most common sign is difficulty breathing.

• When used to decrease clotting function, aspirin can be given at a low dose once a week. This helps to minimize the risk of NSAID toxicity, even with long-term use.

• Aspirin should be avoided or very carefully monitored in horses with bleeding disorders, liver disease, kidney disease, or GI problems.

• Because of aspirin's effects on clotting function, it should be avoided within two weeks of surgery.

• Overdoses of aspirin can cause GI ulcers, protein loss, and kidney and liver damage. Early signs of toxicity include loss of appetite and depression.

Drug Interactions

• Aspirin should not be combined with other anti-inflammatory drugs that tend to cause GI ulcers, such as corticosteroids and other NSAIDs.

• Aspirin should not be combined with anticoagulant drugs, particularly coumarin derivatives such as warfarin.

• Furosemide will slow down the excretion of aspirin via the kidneys.

Special Considerations

• Aspirin tablets are measured in grains rather than milligrams or grams. One grain equals 64.8 mg.

• Some veterinarians may use more than one NSAID in combination, for example aspirin and phenylbutazone given together. This is sometimes called stacking. Although there is little experimental evidence to support this practice, the theory is that different NSAIDs may act differently on different body systems. Particular care needs to be taken in this situation to avoid additive toxicity.

• Aspirin has a different mechanism of action on blood clotting than do the other NSAIDs, and its effects on blood clotting last much longer than other NSAIDs.

• Aspirin is such an old drug that its use predates the FDA approval process. Aspirin is not a prescription drug.

Special Populations

Breeding Animals

Aspirin has been shown to delay labor and delivery in other species. It is generally not recommended in pregnant animals, particularly in late pregnancy. No information on aspirin's effect on sperm production was found. Aspirin should only be used in breeding animals when the benefits outweigh the potential risks.

Foals

Aspirin may be used in foals, but it should be used with particular caution and attention to potential GI ulceration and kidney function. Nursing foals may metabolize or excrete aspirin more slowly than adult horses. Premature foals, septicemic foals, foals with questionable kidney or liver function, and foals with diarrhea require careful monitoring. Drugs to protect the GI tract such as omeprazole, cimetidine, or sucralfate are frequently used with NSAIDs.

Ponies

Pony breeds may be more susceptible to side effects from NSAIDs than horses. When NSAIDs are used in ponies, they should be used with caution and at the lowest effective dose.

Geriatrics

Older horses and especially those with decreased kidney or liver function may be more at risk for side effects from NSAIDs. When aspirin is used in older horses, it should be used carefully and at the lowest effective dose.

Competition Horses

Aspirin is either a regulated or prohibited substance in most sanctioned competition. USEF has a lengthy discussion of NSAIDs in its drug rules. Aspirin and some of its related byproducts are normally found in horse urine, and many regulatory agencies have a detection threshold for this drug. Aspirin may be detected in urine samples for 24 hours or more, depending on the sensitivity of the test. Its metabolism can vary among horses.

Dose and Route of Administration

Oral: 4.5 to 45 mg/lb, twice a day for pain. Provide less frequent administration to decrease blood clot formation.

Dose Form: Oral boluses (large soft tablets): 60 grain (3.89 grams) and 240 grain (15.55 grams)

AT A GLANCE:

ATROPINE

GENERIC NAME
Atropine

COMMON BRAND NAME
Generics

DRUG TYPE
Anticholinergic

INDICATIONS
Bronchospasm, heart arrhythmias, organophosphate poisoning

Basic Information

Atropine is a purified form of the natural plant alkaloid belladonna, which is present in deadly nightshade (*Atropa belladonna*). The medicinal and poisonous properties of belladonna have been known for many centuries.

Atropine counteracts the effects of the chemical messenger and neurotransmitter acetylcholine by competing for the receptors on sensitive muscle cells. Sensitive muscle cells are primarily the ones not under conscious control in the intestines, heart, sweat glands, lungs, eyes, and urinary system. Horses are relatively resistant to orally administered atropine, but respond to the drug administered by injection.

Veterinarians use injectable atropine in horses for certain types of emergencies. It can be used for bronchodilation in horses having difficulty breathing during acute episodes of heaves or chronic obstructive pulmonary disease (COPD). It is used to treat abnormal heart rhythms, especially when the heart is beating more slowly than normal. This can occur during anesthesia or in response to some other drugs. It is used to treat poisoning or overdose with organophosphates. Some of the older types of dewormers and some fly sprays and other insecticides contain organophosphates.

Atropine is used topically on the eye to dilate the pupil, either for examination or as a part of treatment. For example, it is used in recurrent uveitis or moon blindness where pain causes the pupil to constrict. Dilating the pupil decreases the pain and helps prevent the formation of restrictive scars or adhesions that can permanently interfere with normal pupil function.

Side Effects, Precautions, and Overdose

• Systemic atropine produces a wide range of side effects that are generally dose related.

• Some common side effects of systemic atropine include increased heart and respiratory rates, dry mouth and mucous membranes, slowing of gastrointestinal (GI) motility, abdominal pain, and dilation of the pupil.

• Horses are particularly susceptible to slowing of the GI tract and developing colic due to atropine use.

• Atropine should not be used to treat shock, certain heart conditions, and most GI problems, including colic and diarrheas. Horses with kidney or liver disease are particularly susceptible to side effects.

• Overdose increases the severity of the already mentioned side effects. In addition, restlessness, muscular tremors, loss of coordination, convulsions, and respiratory depression ending in death can occur.

Drug Interactions

• Atropine interacts with a long list of other drugs, including antihistamines, phenothiazine tranquilizers, and some painkillers.

• Long-term corticosteroid use to treat a horse with COPD, for example, can increase the likelihood of side effects from atropine.

Special Considerations

• Atropine was once used as a treatment for gas or spasmodic colic because it slowed the GI tract. It was found in some over-the-counter patent medicinal products. There are safer and more effective drugs available to treat colic.

• In some particularly sensitive individuals, even ophthalmic atropine is sufficient to slow the GI tract and cause motility problems.

• Atropine is a powerful and important drug in veterinary medicine. Despite a long list of warnings, when used under the correct circumstances, it can turn an emergency situation around.

• Atropine is FDA approved in the horse and is a prescription drug. U.S. federal law restricts this drug to use by or on the lawful written or oral order of a licensed veterinarian within the context of a valid veterinarian-client-patient relationship.

Special Populations

Breeding Animals

Atropine crosses the placenta and is found in the milk of other species. No specific information was found regarding atropine use in breeding stallions. The risks and benefits should be considered before using.

Foals

Atropine should be used with extreme caution in foals.

Ponies

Some references state that ponies may be more sensitive to adverse effects of atropine than horses. Atropine should be used with extreme caution in ponies and possibly at a lower dose.

Geriatrics

Atropine should be used with extreme caution in older horses. Horses with kidney or liver disease are particularly susceptible to side effects.

Competition Horses

Atropine is prohibited in most sanctioned competitions. USEF has provisions in its rules for the therapeutic use of prohibited substances. It is important to check with the individual regulatory group.

Dose and Route of Administration

Injectable: 0.005 to 0.05 mg/lb, IV, IM, or subcutaneously. Higher doses are used for organophosphate poisoning.

Dose Form: 0.5 mg/ml, 2 mg/ml, 15 mg/ml

AT A GLANCE:

BISMUTH SUBSALICYLATE

GENERIC NAME
Bismuth subsalicylate

COMMON BRAND NAME
Pepto-Bismol, BismuKote, BismuPaste, Corrective Mixture

DRUG TYPE
Antidiarrheal

INDICATIONS
Diarrhea

Basic Information

Bismuth subsalicylate is frequently used to provide symptomatic relief from diarrhea in foals and in adult horses. Just like in humans, it is used to soothe and protect the gastrointestinal tract. The bismuth in the compound is thought to have some weak antibacterial properties and may provide limited protection from the absorption of toxins. The salicylate component has weak antiprostaglandin activity, which may decrease inflammation and secretion.

Diarrhea in horses can range from mild and transient to full-blown, life-threatening colitis. Maintaining hydration and minimizing the absorption of bacterial endotoxins are frequently the keys to a successful outcome. Some serious cases of diarrhea are not responsive to antibiotics and are treated solely with supportive care while others require appropriate antibiotic therapy. Many horses with diarrhea require intravenous fluids. Diarrhea in horses and foals should always be taken very seriously because of the possibility of dehydration and laminitis. A veterinarian should be consulted in all cases of diarrhea in a horse.

Side Effects, Precautions, and Overdose

• Bismuth subsalicylate is very safe. Darkening of feces and constipation can occur in foals.

• The salicylate portion of bismuth subsalicylate is related to aspirin and theoretically could increase clotting time. This would be very unusual.

• Overdosing with bismuth subsalicylate is very difficult, particularly in the adult horse.

Drug Interactions

• Bismuth subsalicylate is related to aspirin. Care should be taken if both drugs are used concurrently because the risk of side effects is increased.

• Bismuth subsalicylate can decrease the absorption of oral tetracycline antibiotics (doxycycline). If they are being used at the same time, dosing should be separated by at least two hours.

Special Considerations

• Bismuth subsalicylate in combination with other drugs is sometimes used in people for the management of ulcers. There are many more effective and more convenient medications available for the treatment of ulcers in horses. (See Omeprazole, Cimetidine and Ranitidine, Sucralfate.)

• Bismuth subsalicylate is not usually effective for the treatment of abdominal pain or colic.

• Bismuth subsalicylate is generally administered to adult horses via a nasogastric tube because of the large volume of drug required.

• Bismuth subsalicylate is not a prescription drug. Veterinary preparations are available in gallons and are frequently cheaper than purchasing pints of the human product at the drug store.

Special Populations

Breeding Animals

No information was found on the safety of bismuth subsalicylate compounds in breeding animals. As with most drugs, this product should only be used when the benefits outweigh the potential risks.

Foals

Bismuth subsalicylate is commonly used in foals. It is frequently the only treatment necessary for mild foal heat scours.

Ponies

Pony breeds do not appear to differ from horses in their response to bismuth subsalicylate.

Geriatrics

Bismuth subsalicylate should be safe in older horses.

Competition Horses

Bismuth subsalicylate is related to aspirin, which is frequently a regulated drug. Many regulatory groups have a detection threshold for salicylate. It is important to check with the individual regulatory agency, particularly regarding detection times.

Dose and Route of Administration

Oral: Adults: 1 to 2 liters/1,000 lbs, twice a day. Some clinicians may give more often.

Foals: 2 to 6 oz, every six to eight hours

Dose Form: suspension or weight calibrated paste syringe

66 ♦ UNDERSTANDING EQUINE MEDICATIONS

AT A GLANCE:
BUTORPHANOL

GENERIC NAME
Butorphanol tartrate

COMMON BRAND NAME
Torbugesic, Dolorex

DRUG TYPE
Narcotic pain reliever

INDICATIONS
Pain relief

Basic Information

Butorphanol is a synthetic narcotic primarily used for pain relief in the horse. It may be used alone for pain relief or combined with tranquilizers such as xylazine, detomidine, and other drugs for increased pain relief and for making an animal easier and safer to handle. These combinations provide sufficient sedation and pain control for many veterinary procedures, including some types of surgery.

Butorphanol is more than five times more effective in controlling pain than morphine, the classic narcotic drug. Studies show that butorphanol starts to alleviate pain within 15 minutes of administration and generally lasts for about four hours. It is usually given by injection in the muscle (IM) or in the vein (IV).

Side Effects, Precautions, and Overdose

• The most common side effects are temporary loss of coordination and/or sedation. Some horses may show temporary central nervous system excitement, including head tossing, continuous walking, or head pressing.

• Rare side effects, which are usually associated with overdosing, include falling, muscle twitching, seizures, salivation, and constipation.

• With any form of sedation, horses can react suddenly and unexpectedly. Always work carefully around a sedated horse no matter how "asleep" it may appear.

• It is important to keep accurate records of butorphanol and other medications used to treat a horse with colic, particularly if the animal is referred to an equine hospital for intensive care or surgery.

• Butorphanol has a wide margin of safety. Narcotic antagonists such as naloxone may be used in case of accidental overdose.

Drug Interactions

• Butorphanol has additive effects when used with other sedatives, narcotics, antihistamines, and central nervous system depressants. Such combinations cause increased sedation and loss of coordination. The doses of one or more of these drugs may require adjustments if they are used together.

Special Considerations

• Butorphanol is FDA approved in the horse. It is a prescription drug and a controlled substance. U.S. federal law restricts this drug to use by or on the lawful written or oral order of a licensed veterinarian within the context of a valid veterinarian-client-patient relationship.

Special Populations

Breeding Animals

There are no well-controlled studies using butorphanol in breeding mares and stallions. Butorphanol crosses the placenta, and it is also excreted in the milk of lactating mares. There is no indication that the drug causes birth defects, but the manufacturer recommends that it not be used in pregnant animals. The risks and benefits should be carefully considered before using.

Foals

There are no well-controlled studies of butorphanol in foals. It should be used with care and only if the benefits outweigh the risks.

Ponies

Pony breeds do not appear to differ from horses in their response to butorphanol.

Geriatrics

In older people, and those with liver or kidney disease, the initial recommended dose is half the normal dose, and the interval between doses is increased. This work has not been repeated in the horse but may be a reasonable precaution because butorphanol is metabolized and excreted by these organs.

Competition Horses

Butorphanol is a prohibited substance in most sanctioned competitions. It is a prohibited class A medication under the new FEI rules. USEF has provisions in its rules for the therapeutic use of prohibited substances. It is important to check with the individual regulatory group.

Dose and Route of Administration

Injectable: 0.005 to 0.05 mg/lb, IV or IM. There is a wide dose range because this drug is used in combination with other drugs and for different purposes.

Dose Form: 10 mg/ml, injectable

AT A GLANCE:

CEFTIOFUR

GENERIC NAME
Ceftiofur

COMMON BRAND NAME
Naxcel

DRUG TYPE
Antibiotic

INDICATIONS
Susceptible bacterial
infections

Basic Information

Ceftiofur is a newer drug in the class of cephalosporin antibiotics. It is used in horses primarily for the treatment of respiratory disease, but may also be used whenever a broad-spectrum antibiotic is desired.

Cephalosporins kill bacteria by disrupting construction of the bacterial cell wall. This allows cephalosporins to kill only bacteria that are growing, and, therefore, the drug should not be used with bacteriostatic antibiotics that merely prevent or slow bacterial growth. Ceftiofur is a third-generation cephalosporin and is effective against many different bacteria, including both Gram-positive and Gram-negative bacteria. Ceftiofur may be given in the muscle (IM) or intravenously (IV). It is excreted by the kidneys, and very high levels of this antibiotic are present in urine.

Side Effects, Precautions, and Overdose

• Ceftiofur is generally a very safe antibiotic. Side effects are rare at normal doses.

• The most common side effects for ceftiofur are local pain and swelling at the injection site from intramuscular administration. These reactions usually respond to hot compresses and NSAIDs. Contact your veterinarian if you notice a reaction.

• Antibiotic-induced diarrhea has been reported with ceftiofur use. Some veterinarians think that this may be dose-related or that certain populations of horses (young racehorses) are more susceptible.

• Ceftiofur should not be used in patients with previous hypersensitivity to cephalosporins or penicillin antibiotics.

• Not for human use. Cephalosporins and penicillins can cause allergic reactions in certain individuals. People who are allergic to penicillin may have a similar reaction to cephalosporins. Persons with known hypersensitivity to either of these drugs should avoid exposure to this product.

• High doses or overdose of ceftiofur given during safety studies caused diarrhea, colic, and loss of appetite.

Drug Interactions

• Cephalosporins are not recommended with bacteriostatic antibiotics such as chloramphenicol.

Special Considerations

• Antibiotic-induced diarrheas are very serious and can be life threatening. If diarrhea should occur while an animal is on ceftiofur or any other antibiotic, the drug should be discontinued immediately. Aggressive supportive therapy for the diarrhea may be necessary. The manufacturer states that horses under stress may be more prone to ceftiofur-induced diarrhea.

• Ceftiofur is FDA approved in the horse and is a prescription drug. U.S. federal law restricts this drug to use by or on the lawful written or oral order of a licensed veterinarian within the context of a valid veterinarian-client-patient relationship.

Special Populations

Breeding Animals

Ceftiofur has not been studied in the pregnant mare. In other species cephalosporin antibiotics have been shown to cross the placenta but without documented harm to the fetus. It is not known if ceftiofur is excreted in the milk of mares. No information was found regarding ceftiofur use in breeding stallions.

Foals

Ceftiofur is frequently used in foals. It is considered safe and effective for sensitive infections.

Ponies

Pony breeds do not appear to differ from horses in their response to ceftiofur.

Geriatrics

Ceftiofur is used in older horses. It should be used with care in animals with decreased kidney function.

Competition Horses

Ceftiofur is forbidden in any drug-free competition, but many regulatory groups do not prohibit antibiotics. USEF has provisions in its rules for the therapeutic use of prohibited substances; ceftiofur is not restricted for horses showing under the therapeutic substances rules. It is important to check with the individual regulatory organization.

Dose and Route of Administration

Injectable: 0.5 to 2.0 mg/lb, IV or IM, once or twice a day

Dose Form: Sterile powder in 1 gram and 4 gram vials for reconstitution with sterile water. (Do not use saline.)

AT A GLANCE:

CHLORAMPHENICOL

GENERIC NAME
Chloramphenicol

COMMON BRAND NAME
Generics only

DRUG TYPE
Antibiotic

INDICATIONS
Susceptible bacterial
infections

Basic Information

Chloramphenicol is a broad-spectrum bacteriostatic antibiotic. Bacteriostatic antibiotics work by preventing bacteria from growing or reproducing, in contrast to bactericidal antibiotics which kill the susceptible bacteria. Chloramphenicol is effective against many different types of bacteria, including Gram-positive, Gram-negative, and anaerobic bacteria. It is used to treat bacterial infections such as pleuropneumonia, peritonitis, and abdominal abscesses. It is well absorbed orally and is widely distributed throughout the body. Chloramphenicol reaches high drug concentrations in difficult-to-penetrate areas such as joints, the central nervous system, and the eyes.

One major drawback to chloramphenicol is a rare but very serious health risk for humans who handle this drug. (See Precautions.)

Side Effects, Precautions, and Overdose

• PRECAUTION FOR HUMANS: Rare cases of aplastic anemia may occur in some individuals who are exposed to this drug. For these people, even skin contact can cause permanent damage to the bone marrow. Because this anemia is not reversible, chloramphenicol should only be used when other suitable antibiotics are not available and with extreme caution. Gloves and masks should be worn when handling this drug. This drug should be used in a well-ventilated location. Some veterinarians will not prescribe this drug due to liability concerns.

• Side effects from chloramphenicol are not common in horses. Loss of appetite is the most common side effect.

• Horses may develop a temporary anemia from chloramphenicol. It should not be used in horses with known anemia problems.

• Chloramphenicol is metabolized in the liver. It should be used with care in patients with liver or kidney disease. Dose adjustment or monitoring of antibiotic blood level may be necessary.

Drug Interactions

• Chloramphenicol is not compatible with some other antibiotics. It should not be used with bactericidal antibiotics such as the penicillins and aminoglycosides.

• Chloramphenicol can slow the metabolism of barbiturate anesthetics.

Special Considerations

• Oral chloramphenicol tastes terrible. Loss of appetite is a common management problem in the sick horse.

• Chloramphenicol is not FDA approved in the horse. It is accepted practice to use this drug with appropriate warning and precautions for human handlers. It is a prescription drug. U.S. federal law restricts this drug to use by or on the lawful written or oral order of a licensed veterinarian within the context of a valid veterinarian-client-patient relationship.

Special Populations

Breeding Animals

Chloramphenicol crosses the placenta and is present in milk. It may affect the bone marrow of the fetus. It should only be used in pregnant mares when the benefits clearly outweigh the risks. No information was found on effects on breeding stallions.

Foals

Young foals may have immature kidney or liver function and have difficulty metabolizing chloramphenicol. Particular attention should be paid to liver and kidney function. A lower dose may be indicated.

Ponies

Pony breeds do not appear to differ from horses in their response to chloramphenicol.

Geriatrics

Chloramphenicol may be used in older horses with normal kidney and liver function.

Competition Horses

Chloramphenicol is forbidden in any drug-free competition, but many regulatory groups do not prohibit antibiotics. USEF has provisions in its rules for the therapeutic use of prohibited substances; chloramphenicol is not restricted for horses showing under the therapeutic substance rules. It is important to check with the individual regulatory organization.

Dose and Route of Administration

Oral: Foal: 2 to 5 mg/lb, three to four times a day

Adult: 12 to 25 mg/lb, three to four times a day

Injectable: 12 mg/lb, IV or IM, three to four times a day

Dose Form: tablets or capsules, 100 mg, 250 mg, 500 mg, 1,000 mg

AT A GLANCE:

CIMETIDINE AND RANITIDINE

GENERIC NAME
Cimetidine
Ranitidine

COMMON BRAND NAME
Tagamet
Zantac

DRUG TYPE
Histamine H_2 receptor antagonist

INDICATIONS
Ulcers of the gastrointestinal tract, melanoma

Basic Information

Cimetidine and ranitidine are anti-ulcer medications called histamine H_2 receptor antagonists. These drugs prevent the stomach from producing acid. Other commonly used drugs for the management and prevention of equine gastric ulcers are omeprazole and sucralfate.

Equine gastric ulcers have many causes, including diet, medications, stress, or a combination of factors. The location of the ulcers within the stomach and upper gastrointestinal tract may vary and affects which medication is most likely to be effective. Our knowledge of the diagnosis and treatment of equine gastric ulcers has exploded in the last 10 years, primarily due to increased endoscopic examination of the stomach. Foals and racehorses are two populations with a higher risk for gastric ulcers.

Cimetidine can be used as a treatment for melanoma, either alone or in combination with surgery or immunotherapy. Recommended duration of treatment is three months or more.

Side Effects, Precautions, and Overdose

• Cimetidine and ranitidine are considered very safe drugs with few side effects. They should be used with caution or at a reduced dose in horses with decreased liver or kidney function.

• Overdoses of cimetidine are associated with breathing difficulties and heart rhythm disturbances, but little else is known. No information was found on overdose of ranitidine in horses or other animals. Both drugs have a wide margin of safety in laboratory animals.

Drug Interactions

• Cimetidine slows the metabolism of other drugs that are metabolized by the liver, including some cardiac drugs, benzodiazepines, some anticonvulsants, and some antibiotics such as metronidazole.

• Some veterinarians recommend separating oral doses of histamine H_2 receptor antagonists from antacids, metoclopramide, and sucralfate.

• Histamine H_2 receptor antagonists may affect blood clotting in animals on warfarin.

Special Considerations

• Histamine H_2 receptor antagonist drugs are sometimes prescribed as a precaution with nonsteroidal anti-inflammatory drugs (NSAIDs), corticosteroids, and other drugs that can cause stomach ulcers.

• After a positive diagnosis of ulcers, these drugs are usually prescribed for two to three weeks in order to give the ulcers time to heal.

• While histamine H_2 receptor antagonists may improve clinical signs of ulcers in racehorses, some research shows that their ulcers may not heal if the horses remain in training. Omeprazole seems to result in better healing in these horses.

• Cimetidine and ranitidine are not FDA approved in the horse, but they are commonly used and considered accepted practice. They are prescription drugs. U.S. federal law restricts these drugs to use by or on the lawful written or oral order of a licensed veterinarian within the context of a valid veterinarian-client-patient relationship.

Special Populations

Breeding Animals

Histamine H_2 receptor antagonists cross the placenta. Although studies in pregnant laboratory animals show no harm to the developing fetus, there are no studies in horses. These drugs are also excreted in the milk of other species.

No information was available on either drug's use in breeding stallions. In other species, no effect on sperm characteristics was seen.

Foals

Cimetidine and ranitidine are commonly used in foals. Young foals with immature kidney or liver function may have difficulty metabolizing these drugs. Particular attention should be paid to their liver and kidney function and a lower dose may be indicated.

Ponies

There are no specific contraindications to cimetidine and ranitidine use in ponies.

Geriatrics

Histamine H_2 receptor antagonist metabolism is decreased in elderly human patients, especially those with kidney or liver disease. It should be used with caution in older animals, and the dose will usually need to be decreased.

Competition Horses

Cimetidine and ranitidine are forbidden in any drug-free competition. Individual regulatory groups may have permissible detection levels, and detection time may vary, depending on the test used. Some veterinarians use a four-day withdrawal and others use a seven-day withdrawal for cimetidine. No information on ranitidine detection time was found. The FEI now permits histamine H_2 receptor antagonists. USEF has provisions in its rules for the therapeutic use of prohibited substances; these drugs are permitted for horses showing under the therapeutic substance rules. It is important to check with a knowledgeable veterinarian and the individual regulatory group.

Dose and Route of Administration

Oral: Cimetidine: 8 mg/lb, three times a day

Ranitidine: 3 mg/lb, three times a day

Injectable:

Cimetidine: 3 mg/lb, IV, four times a day

Ranitidine: 0.7 mg/lb, IV, three times a day

Dose Form:

Cimetidine HCL injectable: 150 mg/ml

Cimetidine tablets: 200 mg, 300 mg, 400 mg, and 800 mg

Ranitidine injectable: 25 mg/ml

Ranitidine tablets: 75 mg, 150 mg, and 300 mg

AT A GLANCE:

CLENBUTEROL

GENERIC NAME
Clenbuterol

COMMON BRAND NAME
Ventipulmin

DRUG TYPE
Bronchodilator

INDICATIONS
Bronchospasm, chronic obstructive pulmonary disease, respiratory distress

Basic Information

Clenbuterol is a newer bronchodilator used for the management of chronic obstructive pulmonary disease (COPD) and allergic airway disease. Bronchodilators are used in horses to relax smooth muscle surrounding the airways in the lungs and open those airways. Clenbuterol also helps the body clear the lungs and airways by loosening excess mucus.

COPD, frequently called "heaves," is an inflammatory disease of the lungs in horses that causes the small airways to constrict and become clogged with mucus. COPD is a progressive disease, which means that horses with COPD are managed, not cured. It is best treated through a combination of husbandry changes and medication. Bronchodilators and corticosteroids are two of the mainstay medications used in the management and treatment of COPD. Husbandry changes include reducing exposure to the dust in hay and barns and to high ammonia concentrations from urine in poorly ventilated stalls.

Bronchodilators are also sometimes used as performance-enhancing drugs, especially in racehorses. The thought behind their use as performance enhancers is that bronchodilation will improve the horse's oxygen uptake to the blood and muscles.

Side Effects, Precautions, and Overdose

• Side effects are less likely with clenbuterol than with other bronchodilators. They include increased heart rate, trembling, excitement, and sweating.

- Side effects are dose related and rarely seen at lower doses.
- Clenbuterol should not be used in horses with heart problems because it increases heart rate.
- Clenbuterol has been used illegally by some people, including body-builders who are trying to increase their muscle mass.
- Overdose increases the risk and severity of the aforementioned side effects.

Drug Interactions

- Clenbuterol used in combination with other drugs that have a similar mechanism of action increases the risk of cardiovascular side effects.
- Clenbuterol may counteract the effects of prostaglandin and oxytocin on the smooth muscle of the uterus. This drug is used in some countries to prevent premature labor and to decrease uterine contractions during a difficult delivery.

Special Considerations

- Environmental management by limiting exposure to dust and mold is key in controlling COPD. With good environmental management, a lower dose of clenbuterol may be effective.
- Clenbuterol is FDA approved in horses, and it is a prescription drug. U.S. federal law restricts this drug to use by or on the lawful written or oral order of a licensed veterinarian within the context of a valid veterinarian-client-patient relationship.

Special Populations

Breeding Animals

Safety in broodmares and breeding stallions has not been established. Clenbuterol should not be used in late pregnancy as it may interfere with normal labor.

Foals

Clenbuterol is occasionally used in sick foals in respiratory distress due to pneumonia.

Ponies

Pony breeds do not appear to differ from horses in their response to clenbuterol.

Geriatrics

Clenbuterol is relatively safe in older animals without other medical conditions that increase the risk of side effects.

Competition Horses

Clenbuterol is prohibited or regulated in most sanctioned competitions. It is a prohibited class A medication under the new FEI rules. Detection time is affected by the number of doses and the sensitivity of the test. It is possible to detect clenbuterol for as long as 30 days using a very sensitive test. Some state racing commissions are moving toward a withdrawal period of either 72 or 96 hours. Check with the individual regulatory group.

Dose and Route of Administration

Oral: 0.4 microgram (ug)/lb (0.5 ml/100 lbs bodyweight), twice a day for three days. If there is no improvement, the package insert describes a gradually increasing dose program. Therapy should be continued for 30 days. See package insert.

Dose Form: Oral syrup, 72.5 ug/ml

AT A GLANCE:

CORTICOSTEROIDS

GENERIC NAME	COMMON BRAND NAME
Betamethasone	Betasone
Dexamethasone	Azium
Flumethasone	Flucort
Isoflupredone acetate	Predef 2x
Methylprednisolone acetate	Depo-Medrol
Prednisone, Prednisolone	Solu-Delta-Cortef
Triamcinolone	Vetalog

DRUG TYPE	INDICATIONS
Steroid hormone	Anti-inflammatory, immunosuppressive

Basic Information

Corticosteroids are hormones normally produced by the adrenal gland. They are essential for life and affect every level of metabolism and the function of all cells and organ systems. There are two major types of hormones produced by the adrenal gland: mineralocorticoids and glucocorticoids. Mineralocorticoids primarily control salt and water balance in the body. The glucocorticoids, also called corticosteroids, are important in normal protein, carbohydrate, and fat metabolism and for their role in controlling inflammation. There is some crossover in function between these two groups of hormones. This monograph discusses glucocorticoids or corticosteroids.

In the horse, corticosteroids are given systemically to decrease inflammatory and immune responses. They are also injected into joints to decrease local inflammation. Corticosteroids are extremely powerful hormones and have both strong beneficial effects and a definite potential to cause negative side effects. It is important to have a basic understanding of their pharmacology in order to use them successfully and minimize the side effects. Their anti-inflammatory effects are due to multiple actions at the cellular levels. They stabilize cell membranes, alter the movement of different types of white blood cells, and influence chemical responses to inflammation, including reduction of prostaglandin production.

Corticosteroids are used systemically in high doses in emergencies for anaphylactic reactions, spinal cord trauma, or shock. They are used in lower doses to treat allergic reactions, such as heaves, hives, itching, and inflammatory diseases, such as arthritis. Corticosteroids are sometimes used systemically as a "performance-enhancing drug" because they decrease inflammation, possibly enhance glucose metabolism (there is some debate about this), and may have some mood-elevating properties. Obviously, this use is illegal in most competitive situations.

When corticosteroids are used systemically, the basic rule is to use the preparation with the shortest duration of action, at the lowest dose level, and for the shortest period of time possible. Chronic or inappropriate use of corticosteroids can cause life-threatening hormonal and metabolic changes. These drugs may be given orally, topically, or by injection.

Corticosteroids are frequently injected into the joints of horses. Intra-articular corticosteroids dramatically lower the local inflammatory response in that joint. There has been a great deal of research through the years concerning the local effects of corticosteroids on joint health and the ideal duration of rest/exercise post corticosteroid injection. Despite this research, there are no clear-cut answers, and opinion is still divided on these questions. Corticosteroids should not be injected into any joint without an appropriate clinical work up and diagnostics, including radiographs. Intra-articular corticosteroids have systemic effects because they diffuse from the joint into the general circulation. If the dose injected into the joints is large, systemic adverse reactions are possible.

Corticosteroids are also used topically to treat certain conditions of the skin and eyes. Preparations for topical use may include other active ingredients such as antibiotics, antifungals, or miticides, which kill mites.

There are many different corticosteroids available on the market.

Different medical conditions are treated with different corticosteroid drugs, based on the individual drug's pharmacology (potency, speed of onset, duration of action). A major goal in developing new corticosteroid drugs is to increase the anti-inflammatory effect and reduce their crossover effect on salt and water balance.

Side Effects, Precautions, and Overdose

• Systemic side effects to corticosteroids vary depending on the dose and duration of treatment.

• Administration of corticosteroids, either systemically or intra-articularly, can suppress the body's normal production of these hormones.

• Systemic corticosteroids can mask signs of infection, such as an elevated temperature.

• Corticosteroids suppress immune response. Local immune response in injected joints is decreased, increasing the possibility of a bacterial infection in the joint secondary to injection. Horses receiving systemic corticosteroids may be more susceptible to bacterial or viral infections.

• Corticosteroids can cause laminitis in horses and ponies. Some corticosteroids are thought to be more likely to cause laminitis than others are, but any corticosteroid can cause laminitis.

• Increased urination (polyuria), increased water consumption (polydypsia), and muscle wasting can be seen with prolonged corticosteroid use.

• Corticosteroids can cause or worsen gastric ulcers.

Drug Interactions

• When diuretics such as furosemide are given with corticosteroids, there is an increased risk of electrolyte imbalances due to calcium and potassium losses.

• The immune response to vaccination may be reduced when corticosteroids are given at the same time.

• The risk of gastrointestinal ulcers may be increased if corticosteroids and other drugs prone to causing ulcers such as NSAIDs are given at the same time.

• Corticosteroids should not be given intravenously with fluids containing calcium.

Special Considerations

• Cushing's disease (hyperadrenocorticism) is caused by excess corticosteroid. The most common example of naturally occurring Cushing's disease in the horse occurs with pituitary pars intermedia dysfunction. Addison's disease (hypoadrenocorticism) is caused by insufficient mineralocorticoid and sometimes glucocorticoid. Both of these diseases are potentially fatal and can accidentally occur due to overuse or abrupt withdrawal after a prolonged treatment with corticosteroids.

• The doses of corticosteroids that are used in emergency medicine and the treatment of autoimmune diseases are considerably higher than the doses used under other circumstances.

• The corticosteroids listed in the box on page 83 are FDA approved in the horse and are prescription drugs. U.S. federal law restricts this drug to use by or on the lawful written or oral order of a licensed veterinarian within the context of a valid veterinarian-client-patient relationship.

Special Populations

Breeding Animals

Corticosteroids should be avoided during pregnancy and lactation unless the benefits outweigh the risks. Excessive levels may cause birth defects. Corticosteroids can induce labor in cattle. Although it is not well documented, the drugs may present a similar risk in late-pregnancy mares. Some corticosteroids have been shown to have a negative effect on semen characteristics in other species.

Foals

Corticosteroids should be avoided in young foals because the drugs suppress the immune system. Corticosteroids are sometimes used under special circumstances when the benefits outweigh the risks. If they are used in foals, many veterinarians prescribe anti-ulcer medication at the same time.

Ponies

Pony breeds may be more susceptible to developing laminitis than horses. If corticosteroids are used in ponies, the drugs should be used with special attention to dose and duration.

Geriatrics

Corticosteroids may be used in older horses without other underlying health problems. The drugs should not be used in horses with pituitary pars intermedia dysfunction. These horses may already have high levels of natural corticosteroids and are prone to laminitis and suppressed immune function.

Competition Horses

Corticosteroids are commonly used in competition horses both systemically and intra-articularly. They are forbidden in any drug-free competition. They are a prohibited class A medication under the new FEI rules. Most corticosteroids are forbidden for horses showing under USEF's therapeutic substance rules. The exception is dexamethasone; an explanation of dexamethasone use may be found in the group's drug rules.

Different corticosteroids have different withdrawal times, ranging from 24 hours to as long as 44 days for methylprednisolone. Intra-articular corticosteroids can cause a positive drug test. It is important to consult with the individual regulatory group.

Dose and Route of Administration

The dose of all corticosteroids should be adjusted as needed for the individual to control clinical signs with the minimum dose for as short a time as is possible. Tapering doses are frequently used at the end of a course of corticosteroids.

Oral:

Betamethasone: 0.01 to 0.05 mg/lb

Dexamethasone: 10 mg/day for an adult horse. Maintenance dose for management of COPD will probably be much less.

Flumethasone: 0.001 to 0.004 mg/lb/day

Prednisone: 0.01 to 2.0 mg/lb, twice a day

Triamcinolone: 0.005 to 0.01 mg/lb, twice a day

Injectable:

Betamethasone: 0.01 to 0.05 mg/lb/day, IM. May be used intra-articularly.

Dexamethasone: 0.01 to 0.1 mg/lb or 10 mg/day for an adult horse, IV or IM. The high end of the dose range is for emergency or shock use.

Isoflupredone acetate: 5 to 14 mg/day for an adult horse, IM. May be used intra-articularly.

Methylprednisolone acetate: 0.1 to 0.35 mg/lb for an adult horse, IM. May be used intra-articularly and intralesionally.

Prednisolone sodium succinate: 1 to 2.5 mg/lb, IV, for the treatment of septic shock

Prednisone: 0.01 to 2 mg/lb, IM, twice a day

Triamcinolone: 0.01 to 0.02 mg/lb/day, IM or subcutaneous. May be used intra-articularly and intralesionally.

Dose Form:

Betasone: 7 mg/ml injectable. (This product is a combination of two forms of betamethasone to provide both an immediate and a longer lasting effect.)

Dexamethasone: 2 mg/ml injectable and packets containing 10 mg oral powder

Flumethasone: 0.5 mg/ml

Isoflupredone acetate: 2 mg/ml

Methylprednisolone acetate: 20 mg/ml and 40 mg/ml

Prednisone: 20 and 50 mg tablets

Prednisolone: 10 mg/ml and 50 mg/ml

Triamcinolone: 2 mg/ml or 6 mg/ml or 1.5 mg tablets

AT A GLANCE:

CYPROHEPTADINE

GENERIC NAME
Cyproheptadine

COMMON BRAND NAME
Periactin, formulation
from specialty pharmacies

DRUG TYPE
Antihistamine, antiserotonin

INDICATIONS
Pituitary pars intermedia
dysfunction or "pituitary
adenoma," head shakers

Basic Information

Cyproheptadine is an antihistamine that also has antiserotonin activity. It is used in the treatment of both pituitary pars intermedia dysfunction and head shaking.

For many years pituitary pars intermedia dysfunction was called pituitary adenoma. This is no longer thought to be technically correct. In most cases pituitary pars intermedia dysfunction is caused by enlargement or hypertrophy of the pituitary gland; only rarely is there actually a tumor. Because animals with pituitary pars intermedia dysfunction usually have clinical signs similar to Cushing's disease in humans, this condition may also be called equine Cushing's-like disease (ECD). Regardless of the name, this is a fairly common problem of the older horse or pony.

Cyproheptadine has been used successfully in treating some pituitary problems in humans and dogs. The response in horses is more variable.

When cyproheptadine is used for the treatment of head shakers, it is being used for its antihistamine properties. Head shakers present a troubling medical/behavioral problem, and there are many possible causes. Cyproheptadine is only one of many possible treatments for this frustrating problem. In those cases in which there is an allergic component, it may be of benefit.

Side Effects, Precautions, and Overdose

• Common side effects include sedation, dry mucous membranes, and increased heart rate.

• Overdose causes similar but more severe side effects.

Drug Interactions

• Cyproheptadine may have an additive effect when combined with other central nervous system (CNS) depressant drugs such as tranquilizers.

Special Considerations

• Pergolide is considered the drug of choice for pituitary pars intermedia dysfunction. Cyproheptadine is used in addition to pergolide or occasionally on its own.

• Cyproheptadine has a wide margin of safety. Some veterinarians use higher doses than the doses stated here.

• Although cyproheptadine is not FDA approved for use in horses, it is commonly used and considered accepted practice to do so. It is a prescription drug. U.S. federal law restricts this drug to use by or on the lawful written or oral order of a licensed veterinarian within the context of a valid veterinarian-client-patient relationship.

Special Populations

Breeding Animals

High doses of cyproheptadine have been tested in laboratory animals without causing detectable harm to the fetus. This work has not been done in horses. It is not known if cyproheptadine is excreted in milk. Cyproheptadine should only be used in pregnant or lactating animals if the benefits outweigh the risks. No information was found on cyproheptadine use in breeding stallions.

Foals

No information was found on cyproheptadine use in foals.

Ponies

Pony breeds do not appear to differ from horses in their response to cyproheptadine.

Geriatrics

Cyproheptadine is commonly used in older horses and ponies for the treatment of pituitary adenomas.

Competition Horses

Cyproheptadine is prohibited or regulated in most sanctioned competitions. Oral drugs are much more likely to have variable detection times. Long-term or repeated doses can also affect detection times. USEF has provisions in its rules for the therapeutic use of prohibited substances. Consult your veterinarian and the individual regulatory group if you are competing with a horse receiving cyproheptadine.

Dose and Route of Administration

Oral: 0.12 mg/lb, once a day. Some veterinarians may use higher doses or dose twice a day.

Dose Form: 4 mg tablets, specialty formulations in any concentration

AT A GLANCE:

DESLORELIN

GENERIC NAME
Deslorelin

COMMON BRAND NAME
Ovuplant

DRUG TYPE
Synthetic hormone

INDICATIONS
Induce ovulation in mares

Basic Information

Deslorelin is a synthetic hormone that mimics the action of gonadotropin releasing hormone (GnRH). GnRH is produced in an area of the brain called the hypothalamus and stimulates the release of the pituitary hormones that cause ovulation from mature ovarian follicles. Deslorelin reliably causes ovulation within 36 to 48 hours of administration in 86% of mares with follicles at least 30 mm in diameter. Ideally, this permits the mare to be bred at an optimal time for conception, resulting in fewer breedings per cycle and a higher rate of pregnancy.

Deslorelin has been widely available since 1998 although it was being studied for about 10 years before its commercial release. It is manufactured as an implant that is injected under the skin and releases the drug continually for about 72 hours. There is also an injectable version available with only about 16 to 21 hours of activity. Human chorionic gonadotropin (HCG) is another hormone commonly used to induce ovulation in mares.

Side Effects, Precautions, and Overdose

• Injection site reactions including heat, pain, and local swelling can occur. These reactions usually respond to hot compresses and NSAIDs. Contact your veterinarian if you notice a reaction.

• The manufacturer has reported no systemic reactions based on its safety studies.

• Accidental overdose (multiple injections) could increase the possibility of a prolonged interestrous interval (delayed return to heat) should the mare not become pregnant on that cycle.

Drug Interactions
- No drug interactions were listed in the manufacturer's drug insert.

Special Considerations
- For deslorelin to be effective in inducing ovulation there must be a large or dominant follicle. The manufacturer recommends that deslorelin be used with follicles that are 30 mm or greater in diameter. Follicles that are small or regressing are less likely to ovulate.
- Deslorelin comes packaged in a preloaded syringe with an attached large bore "implanter" or needle. Usually a veterinarian will implant the deslorelin after palpating or ultrasounding the mare to determine that she has a large follicle and is ready to be bred. Directions for implanting the deslorelin are in the package insert. The deslorelin implant is absorbed.
- Because deslorelin has been shown to prolong the interestrous interval for some of the mares that do not get pregnant on that cycle, some veterinarians remove the implant after ovulation in order to decrease the chances of this happening. This can be easily done by implanting the deslorelin in the vulvar mucosa.
- Deslorelin is FDA approved in the horse and it is a prescription drug. U.S. federal law restricts the use of this drug by or on the lawful written or oral order of a licensed veterinarian.

Special Populations
Breeding Animals
Deslorelin is regularly used in non-pregnant broodmares for the management of their heat cycle. No adverse effects on nursing foals have been noted. There are no indicated uses for deslorelin in pregnant mares or in stallions.

Foals

Deslorelin is not indicated for use in foals.

Ponies

Pony breeds are similar to horses in their response to deslorelin.

Geriatrics

Deslorelin has no indications for use in older horses apart from older broodmares.

Competition Horses

Deslorelin would not be commonly used in competition horses because they are not usually also being used as broodmares. It would be forbidden in any drug-free competition, but it may not be regulated under many types of rules. Check with the individual regulatory group.

Dose and Route of Administration

Injectable: one subcutaneous injection of 2.1 mg in a controlled release form per heat cycle

Dose Form: preloaded syringe with large bore needle

AT A GLANCE:

DETOMIDINE HYDROCHLORIDE

GENERIC NAME
Detomidine hydrochloride

COMMON BRAND NAME
Dormosedan

DRUG TYPE
Sedative/analgesic

INDICATIONS
Tranquilization and pain relief

Basic Information

Detomidine is a sedative that also provides significant pain relief. The mechanism of action of detomidine is similar to that of xylazine.

Detomidine is a relatively new tranquilizer and is the strongest of the commonly used tranquilizers. It provides deeper and longer-lasting sedation than xylazine or acepromazine. Detomidine is sometimes used in combination with butorphanol and other drugs for chemical restraint during many veterinary procedures or as a pre-operative drug.

Detomidine may also be used for pain relief, especially in colic cases. Because the level of pain relief provided by detomidine is powerful enough to mask cases of colic that might require surgery, it should not be used without thorough veterinary evaluation.

Side Effects, Precautions, and Overdose

• Detomidine initially slows the heart rate and can change the heart rhythm in some horses (dropped beats).

• Horses will drop their heads and appear very sedate. Moderate loss of coordination, sweating, and increased salivation are common.

• With any form of sedation, horses can react suddenly and unexpectedly. Always work carefully around a sedated horse no matter how "asleep" it may appear.

• Although detomidine provides some pain relief, it does not completely block pain. Horses can and will respond to painful stimulation.

• It is important to keep accurate records of detomidine and other medications used to treat a horse with colic, particularly if the animal is referred to an equine hospital for intensive care or surgery.

• Detomidine should not be used in horses with abnormal heart rhythm, heart disease, respiratory disease, or kidney disease. Detomidine should be used with caution in horses in shock or in horses that are suffering from heat stress or hypothermia.

• According to the manufacturer, detomidine is safe at up to five times the normal dose. Overdose can cause heart arrhythmias, low blood pressure, and respiratory and central nervous system depression.

• Yohimbine is a drug that can be used to reverse some of the effects of detomidine.

Drug Interactions

• Detomidine has additive effects when combined with other sedatives, tranquilizers, and general anesthetic drugs. Although such combinations are frequently used in veterinary practice, only veterinarians experienced with these drugs should do so.

• Detomidine should not be used with intravenous sulfonamide drugs (intravenous trimethoprim/sulfa).

Special Considerations

• When sedating a horse using detomidine, it is important to wait until the drug has taken effect before beginning any procedure. Detomidine is faster acting than other commonly used sedatives. Sedation occurs two to four minutes after intravenous (IV) injection and about five minutes after intramuscular (IM) injection.

• Detomidine is FDA approved in the horse and is a prescription drug. U.S. federal law restricts this drug to use by or on the lawful written or oral order of a licensed veterinarian within the context of a valid veterinarian-client-patient relationship.

Special Populations

Breeding Animals

No information was found regarding safety during pregnancy or lactation. It is not known if detomidine is present in milk. Although stallions may relax and drop their penises when treated with detomidine, there are no reports of penile paralysis such as those with acepromazine.

Foals

Because detomidine can cause a low heart rate and slow breathing, it should be used with caution in sick foals or very young foals. Detomidine can affect an animal's ability to regulate its temperature. If it is used in very young foals, the foal should remain in a temperature-controlled area until it has fully recovered. When detomidine is used in young foals, it is generally used at a lower dose.

Ponies

Pony breeds do not appear to differ from horses in their response to detomidine.

Geriatrics

Detomidine may be used with caution in older animals. When detomidine is used in older horses, it is generally used at a lower dose.

Draft Horses

Draft horse breeds are especially sensitive to most sedatives. When detomidine is used in draft horse breeds, it is generally used at a lower dose.

Competition Horses

Detomidine is a prohibited substance in most sanctioned competitions. It is a prohibited class A medication under the new FEI rules. It may be detected in the blood for approximately 48 hours and in urine for up to 72 hours. Detection may be affected by the number of doses and the sensitivity of the test. USEF has provisions in its rules for the therapeutic use of prohibited substances.

AT A GLANCE:

DICLOFENAC SODIUM

GENERIC NAME
Diclofenac Sodium

COMMON BRAND NAME
Surpass

DRUG TYPE
Nonsteroidal anti-inflammatory drug

INDICATIONS
Pain relief, particularly for osteoarthritis, anti-inflammatory

Basic Information

Diclofenac sodium is a topical nonsteroidal anti-inflammatory (NSAID) cream which is labeled for the treatment of pain and inflammation associated with osteoarthritis in the hock, knee, fetlock, and pastern joints of the horse. It is also commonly used to decrease soft tissue swelling in the lower leg.

Diclofenac sodium uses a new technology called liposome delivery as a means of carrying the drug past the skin to the target tissue. Liposomes provide a "locally enhanced topical delivery" that both enhances the penetration of the drug and also sustains the drug's release at the target tissue. For example, if one applies this drug over the right hock, the major portion of the drug can be found in the tissues around the right hock and less throughout the rest of the body.

Diclofenac sodium is an NSAID so it works via the same mechanisms as other NSAIDs such as phenylbutazone, flunixin meglumine, and ketoprofen. In general, NSAIDs, including diclofenac sodium, decrease inflammation and provide pain relief by inhibiting the body's production of prostaglandin and other mediators of the body's inflammatory response.

Side Effects, Precautions, and Overdose

• Adverse reactions to diclofenac sodium are very uncommon

when the drug is used according to directions.

• Some horses may develop "skin crud" while being treated, particularly if they have long hair on their legs. The cream and environmental dirt builds up over the treated area. This can be avoided by regular washing with mild shampoos.

• As a group, NSAIDs can cause gastric ulceration, diarrhea, colic, and kidney damage. NSAIDs should be avoided or very carefully monitored in horses with liver disease, kidney disease, or gastrointestinal (GI) problems.

• Overdoses of diclofenac sodium cause more severe manifestations of the side effects. Early signs of toxicity include loss of appetite, weight loss, colic, and depression.

Drug Interactions

• Avoid combining with other anti-inflammatory drugs that tend to cause GI ulcers, such as corticosteroids and other NSAIDs.

Special Considerations

• This is a drug, not a hand cream. It is important to wear gloves when using diclofenac sodium. For the same reasons that it crosses the skin in horses, it will also cross the skin in people.

• It is also important to pay attention to the amount of drug applied, the area over which it is applied, and the duration of use. The temptation with a topical product may be to get a little carried away.

• Peak tissue levels of the drug occur from about six hours after administration until about 18 hours after administration.

• Different veterinarians report variable response to diclofenac sodium for pain relief due to osteoarthritis. Some feel it is quite useful and others are not as enthusiastic. This may be at least partially due to case selection.

• Diclofenac sodium is a prescription drug. U.S. federal law restricts the use of this drug by or on the lawful written or oral order of a licensed veterinarian within the context of a valid veterinarian-client-patient relationship. A client information sheet is available to be dispensed with the product.

Special Populations

Breeding Animals

There have been no studies on the safety of this drug in breeding animals.

Foals

Premature foals, septicemic foals, foals with questionable kidney or liver function, and foals with diarrhea require careful monitoring. Drugs to protect the GI tract such as omeprazole, cimetidine, and sucralfate are frequently used with NSAIDs.

Ponies

Pony breeds may be more susceptible to side effects from NSAIDs than horses. Using lower doses should be considered.

Geriatrics

Older horses, especially those with decreased kidney or liver function, may be more susceptible to side effects from NSAIDs. When these drugs are used in older horses, they should be used at the lowest effective dose.

Competition Horses

Diclofenac sodium is either a regulated or prohibited substance in most sanctioned competitions. It is not permitted in any drug-free competition, and it is a prohibited class A medication under the new FEI rules. USEF has a lengthy discussion on the use of NSAIDs, including diclofenac sodium, in its drug rules.

Diclofenac sodium may be detected in urine samples for at least two days depending on the sensitivity of the test. Some regulatory agencies may have a permissible drug level threshold. It is important to check with the individual regulatory group.

Dose and Route of Administration

Topical: Apply a five-inch ribbon twice a day over the affected area for up to 10 days.

Dose Form: Topical cream containing 1% diclofenac sodium

AT A GLANCE:

DIMETHYL SULFOXIDE

GENERIC NAME
Dimethyl sulfoxide, DMSO
Methylsulfonyl methane, MSM

COMMON BRAND NAME
Domoso
Flexagen, Vita-Flex MSM

DRUG TYPE
DMSO: Anti-inflammatory
analgesic vehicle to enhance
absorption of other drugs
MSM: Anti-inflammatory and
analgesic

INDICATIONS
DMSO: Topically for pain
and inflammation,
reduction of swelling;
systemically to reduce
inflammation in a number
of conditions
MSM: arthritis, nonspecif-
ic inflammation

Basic Information

DMSO is a liquid solvent that attracts or absorbs water. It has anti-inflammatory and mild antibacterial properties. Because it is able to penetrate skin and other tissues, it is frequently used to carry other drugs through the skin and into the various tissues of the body.

DMSO is FDA approved only for topical application to skin. However, it is used to treat a number of conditions and administered by several different routes. It is administered systemically for the emergency treatment of brain and spinal cord inflammation caused by trauma, exertional rhabdomyolysis or tying up, endotoxemia, laminitis, and neonatal maladjustment syndrome. When used systemically, it is diluted and administered either by nasogastric tube or by intravenous injection. DMSO can also be diluted in sterile saline to flush infected joints. There are probably few areas of the horse's body that have escaped treatment with DMSO in one form or another.

MSM is a metabolite of DMSO that is used to decrease inflammation and pain. It is available as an oral preparation or dietary supplement. Although there has been a lot of MSM sold and used through the years, there is not much scientific support for its efficacy. It does, however, appear to be safe and non-toxic.

Side Effects, Precautions, and Overdose

• PRECAUTIONS FOR HUMANS: Avoid contact with skin when handling DMSO. Rubber gloves should be worn when using this product. Skin irritation is common. DMSO should be used in well-ventilated areas. Some individuals have more pronounced systemic reactions to DMSO exposure, including mild sedation and drowsiness. For a full description of side effects, read the manufacturer's insert.

• DMSO will carry almost anything across the skin. Care should be exercised that this solvent does not inadvertently carry extraneous or toxic compounds into the body.

• DMSO can cause skin irritation and "blistering" in horses. This skin response is caused by histamine release. Some horses object violently to topical DMSO due to pain or skin irritation while others do not seem to mind.

• When first diluted for systemic use, DMSO causes a chemical reaction releasing heat. The solution should be allowed to cool before tubing or administering intravenously (IV).

• Systemic DMSO should be used very carefully in animals in shock or suffering from dehydration. Appropriate IV fluid therapy may be necessary before and during the administration of DMSO.

• Intravenous DMSO may cause some destruction of red blood cells. This can be partially avoided by slow administration and dilution of the DMSO in IV fluids.

• Overdose of DMSO by systemic administration generally requires large doses, rapid administration, or possibly inadequate dilution. Mild signs of toxicity include sedation and blood in the urine. More serious signs of overdose include difficulty breathing, seizures, coma, and death.

Drug Interactions

• The effects of corticosteroids and atropine may be prolonged or increased by DMSO.

• DMSO should not be used with organophosphates.

Special Considerations

• DMSO is partially excreted through the lungs, causing a characteristic "bad breath" in animals and humans that are exposed to it. Many people liken the smell to onions or garlic, although it really has a characteristic noxious smell all its own.

• When DMSO is used IV, it should be diluted to a 10% to 20% solution.

• In some other species, DMSO can cause changes to the lens of the eye. This is not a common problem in the horse.

• Topical use of DMSO is FDA approved in the horse. Systemic use of DMSO is not FDA approved, though many systemic uses are accepted practice. Medical grade DMSO is a prescription drug. U.S. federal law restricts this drug to use by or on the lawful written or oral order of a licensed veterinarian within the context of a valid veterinarian-client-patient relationship.

• MSM is a feed supplement and is not regulated by the FDA.

Special Populations

Breeding Animals

High doses of DMSO have caused birth defects in some but not all laboratory species that were tested. In light of this mixed evidence, DMSO should only be used in pregnant animals when the benefits outweigh the risks.

Foals

DMSO is sometimes used systemically in emergency medicine on very sick young foals, especially neonatal maladjustment syndrome or "dummy foals." Particular care should be used with topical DMSO on foals, as their skin can be more sensitive than adult skin.

Ponies

Pony breeds do not appear to differ from horses in their response to DMSO.

Geriatrics

Topical DMSO is safe in older horses. Systemic DMSO should be safe if liver and kidney function is normal.

Competition Horses

DMSO is a prohibited substance in any drug-free competition although individual regulatory groups may have permissible detection levels. After oral administration of DMSO, detection times may vary from 36 to 72 hours depending on which testing method is used. It is a prohibited class B medication under the new FEI rules. USEF has provisions in its rules for the therapeutic use of prohibited substances; DMSO is permitted for horses showing under the therapeutic substance rules. It is important to check with the individual regulatory body.

The real issue with topical DMSO is its ability to carry another prohibited substance into the body and inadvertently cause a drug violation.

Dose and Route of Administration

Topical: Apply liberally to skin. Limit to no more than 100 ml/per day for no more than 30 days.

Oral: 0.5 gram/lb diluted to a 10% solution in 5% dextrose or saline. May be repeated.

Injectable: 0.5 gram/lb diluted to a 10% solution in 5% dextrose or saline. May be repeated.

Dose Form: 90% solution (only medical grade DMSO should be used). Gel for topical use.

MSM: Different preparations are manufactured and packaged differently. Follow package directions.

AT A GLANCE:

DIOCTYL SODIUM SULFOSUCCINATE

GENERIC NAME
Dioctyl sodium sulfosuccinate,
DSS

COMMON BRAND NAME
Dioctynate

DRUG TYPE
Stool softener and laxative

INDICATIONS
Impaction colic and
constipation

Basic Information

Dioctyl sodium sulfosuccinate or DSS is a laxative or stool softener that is diluted in water and administered by nasogastric tube (stomach tube) to horses with an intestinal blockage due to fecal impaction. It works by reducing the surface tension of the impaction and permitting water to penetrate and soften the fecal mass. DSS also mildly increases intestinal secretion and intestinal motility, which may aid in its action.

DSS is sometimes diluted and used as an enema for young foals with meconium impactions.

Side Effects, Precautions, and Overdose

• DSS can cause diarrhea and increased abdominal pain, especially at higher doses.

• Treatment with DSS should be spaced by 48 hours. It is generally only given twice.

• Excess fluid accumulation or gastric reflux should be ruled out before oral administration of DSS or any liquid. Horses that have gastric reflux may not be able to propel the fluid forward and may be accumulating fluid in the stomach or small intestine. They are frequently not good candidates for fluids administered by nasogastric tube and may require other diagnostics and treatment.

Drug Interactions

• DSS should not be administered at the same time as mineral oil because its effectiveness might be compromised.

Special Considerations

• The treatment and prognosis for impactions vary with the location in the gastrointestinal tract and severity of the impaction.

• The dose of DSS is not well established. Different veterinarians may use different doses. Higher doses are associated with more frequent and severe side effects.

• DSS is only sold to veterinarians. Only a licensed veterinarian should perform nasogastric tubing.

Special Populations

Breeding Animals

No information was found regarding DSS use in breeding animals.

Foals

DSS may be used in enemas for foals with meconium impactions.

Ponies

Pony breeds do not appear to differ from horses in their response to DSS.

Geriatrics

DSS should be safe to use in older horses.

Competition Horses

No information regarding DSS use in competition horses was found.

Dose and Route of Administration

Oral: In an adult horse 4 to 8 ounces diluted in 8 liters of water

Dose Form: 5% solution, which also contains water and propylene glycol

AT A GLANCE:

DOMPERIDONE

GENERIC NAME
Domperidone

COMMON BRAND NAME
Equidone

DRUG TYPE
Dopamine receptor antagonist

INDICATIONS
Prevention and treatment of fescue toxicosis in pregnant mares

Basic Information

Domperidone is a new treatment for fescue toxicosis in pregnant mares. Fescue toxicosis is a very serious health and management problem in parts of the world where endophyte-infected fescue grass is found in and around the pastures. This includes most of the continental United States although clinical problems are especially prevalent in the South.

Fescue toxicosis is caused by a fungal endophyte (internal plant fungus) called *Neotyphodium coenophialum* that grows in fescue. Millions of acres of pasture in the United States contain endophyte-infected fescue. Endophyte-infected fescue is an aggressive grass and has been know to overrun established stands of other grasses. Toxins produced by the endophyte depress prolactin and progesterone, which are important hormones for normal labor, delivery, and lactation. The toxins depress these hormones by increasing the activity of dopamine, an important neurotransmitter and chemical messenger produced by the nervous system. Domperidone counteracts the effects of the fungal toxins by competitively blocking dopamine receptors.

Mares with fescue toxicosis have increased gestation lengths; poor or no udder development; low milk production or agalactia (no milk production); a high incidence of premature placental separation (red bag) or retained placenta; thick or abnormal placentas; difficult deliveries (dystocia); large, weak, and/or dysmature foals; and increased foal and mare mortality.

Side Effects, Precautions, and Overdose

• Leakage of milk or colostrum prior to foaling has been reported as a side effect. This can be managed by collecting and banking colostrum or by reducing the dosage level once leaking occurs.

• Domperidone may cause a false-positive reading on the milk calcium test that is used to predict foaling.

• Domperidone should not be used whenever the stimulation of gastrointestinal (GI) motility might be dangerous for example in the presence of GI hemorrhage, mechanical obstruction, or perforation.

• No information regarding overdose was found.

Drug Interactions

• No studies of drug interactions have been performed in the horse at this time.

• Antacids and antisecretory drugs should not be given at the same time as domperidone. Because domperidone affects gastric motility, it may influence the absorption of other oral drugs.

Special Considerations

• Not all fescue is infected with the endophyte *Neotyphodium coenophialum*. Consult with your veterinarian regarding the incidence of fescue toxicity in your area. Testing of the pasture can be arranged.

• Domperidone can be used for other non-fescue related agalactia and low milk production.

• Prior to the use of domperidone, the best management technique available for fescue toxicosis was the removal of pregnant mares from pasture 60 to 90 days prior to delivery. Domperidone offers a treatment alternative.

• Feed supplementation with vitamin E and selenium are not effective in preventing or treating fescue toxicosis.

• Recent research shows that domperidone may be used to promote follicular development in the transitional mare and to induce lactation in barren or maiden mares.

• Domperidone is under patent and has been approved in other countries. It is not yet FDA approved in the United States, but it is in the homestretch of the approval process. It is a prescription drug and may be purchased by a veterinarian through the manufacturer. U.S. federal law restricts the use of this drug by or on the lawful written or oral order of a licensed veterinarian.

Special Populations

Breeding Animals

Domperidone is used in pregnant mares when fescue toxicosis is diagnosed or suspected. It may be continued after foaling to aid in milk production.

Foals

Domperidone is not used in foals.

Ponies

Pony breeds do not appear to differ from horse breeds in their response to domperidone.

Geriatrics

Domperidone is not used in older horses with the exception of pregnant mares for the purposes discussed above.

Competition Horses

Domperidone is not used in competition horses. It would be prohibited in any drug free competition, but no other competition information was available. Consult with the individual regulatory agency.

Dose and Route of Administration

Oral: Prior to foaling for suspected fescue toxicosis: 0.5 mg/lb once a day starting at least 10 to 15 days prior to foaling date. May continue for five to 10 days after foaling if milk production is inadequate.

Dose Form: Multi-dose oral syringe containing 110 mg/domperidone per ml of gel

AT A GLANCE:

ENROFLOXACIN

GENERIC NAME
Enrofloxacin

COMMON BRAND NAME
Baytril

DRUG TYPE
Fluroquinolone Antibiotic

INDICATIONS
Susceptible bacterial
infections

Basic Information

Enrofloxacin is a broad spectrum bactericidal antibiotic. Although the mechanism of action is not well understood, enrofloxacin is effective against a broad spectrum of Gram-positive and Gram-negative bacteria. It is not effective against anaerobic bacteria and may be variable against *Streptococcus* infections.

Enrofloxacin is well absorbed orally and can be given once a day. This makes it a very attractive antibiotic choice for difficult to treat infections, particularly those that need long-term antibiotics. Some examples might be osteomyelitis, sinus infections, difficult soft tissue infections, peritonitis, and pleuritis or pneumonia.

Side Effects, Precautions, and Overdose

• Enrofloxacin and the other fluroquinolone antibiotics can cause developmental cartilage abnormalities. As a consequence most veterinarians try to avoid these drugs in young horses.

• Animals with severe kidney or liver problems may need a reduced dose of enrofloxacin. Hydration should be monitored and fluid therapy used in animals at risk for dehydration.

• Enrofloxacin should be used with caution or avoided in animals at risk for seizures. This drug is not used in humans due to central nervous system stimulation.

• Enrofloxacin should not be used for regional antibiotic perfusion because it is too irritating and will cause vasculitis.

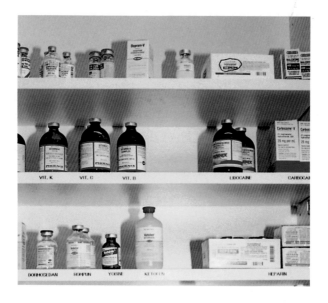

Many equine medications are prescription
drugs and must be dispensed by a veterinarian.
Below, a veterinarian dispenses oral
medications to a client.

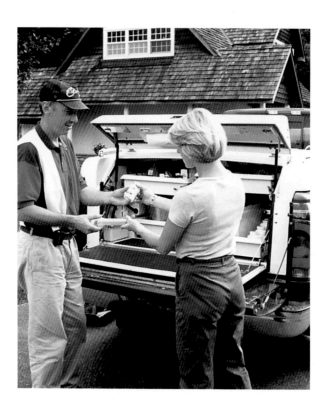

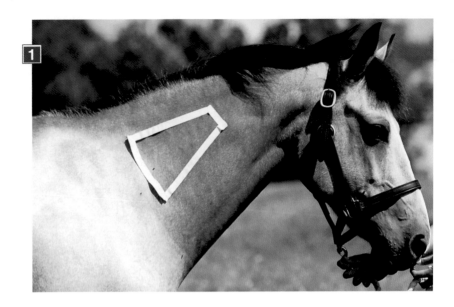

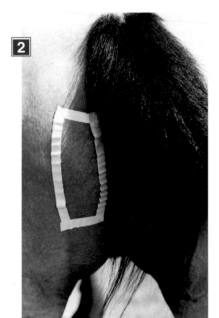

Sites for injections are easily identified for the neck (1), hind leg (2), and gluteals (3).

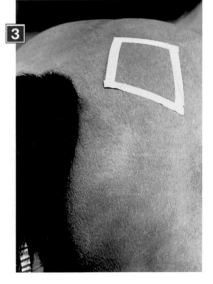

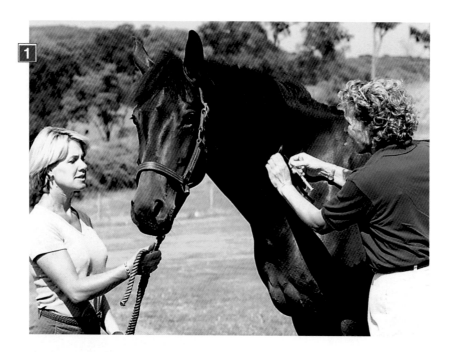

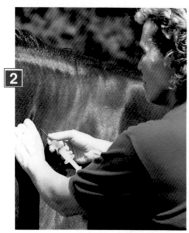

An intramuscular injection
in the neck (1 & 2)
and injecting in the hind leg (3).

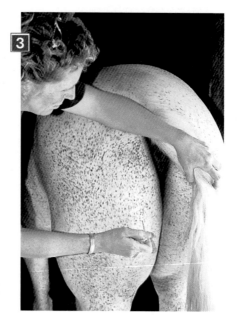

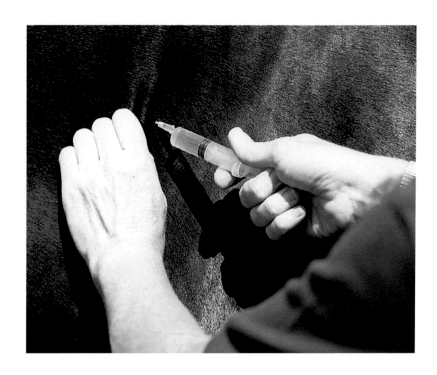

When giving an IM injection, always be sure to
draw back and check for blood (above)
before administering the medication.

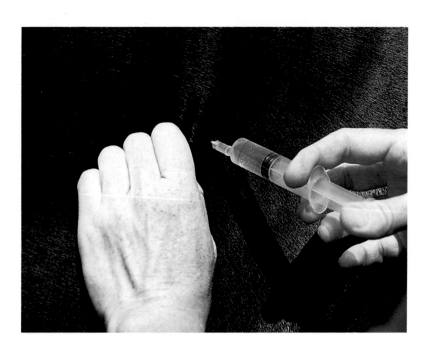

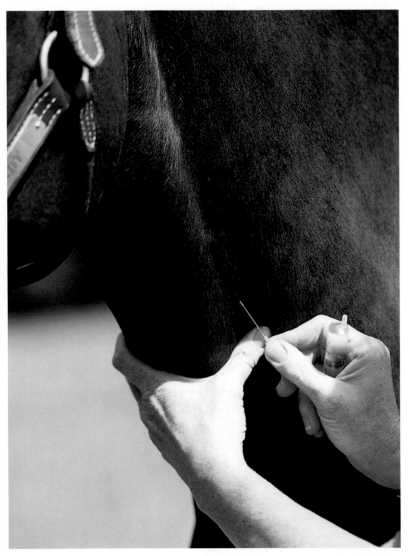

Proper placement of a needle for an intravenous injection.

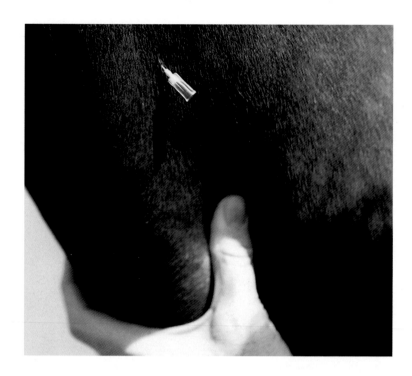

A needle in the jugular vein (top) and
aspirating blood to check placement of the needle.

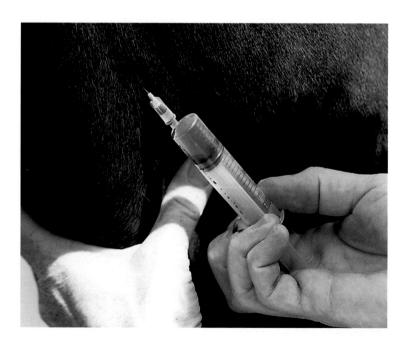

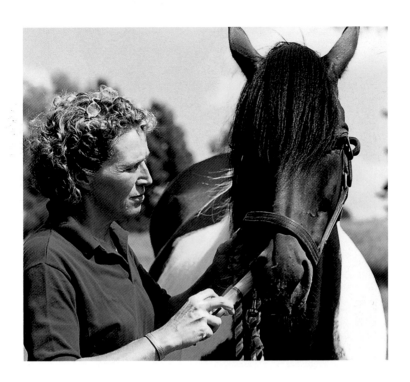

Dosing with an oral medication. Keeping the horse's head aloft can prevent him from spitting out the medication.

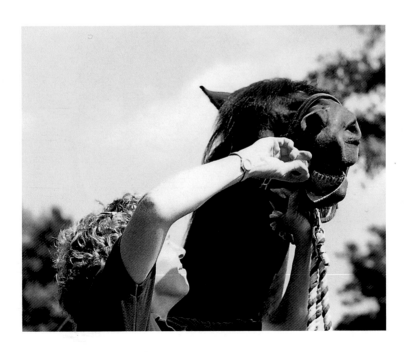

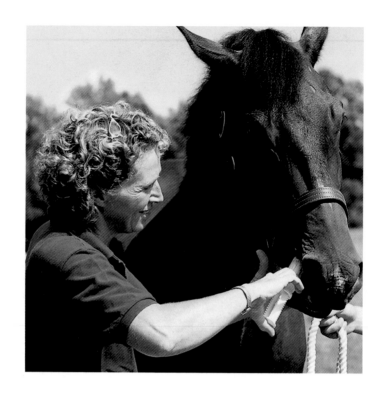

Dosing with paste.

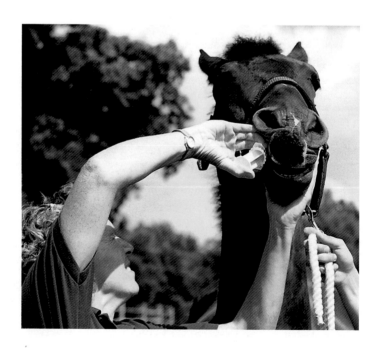

- Oral enrofloxacin can cause mucous membrane irritation, redness, slobbering, and swelling.
- A single overdose is unlikely to cause toxicity. In dogs given 10 times the normal dose, adverse effects were limited to loss of appetite and vomiting. There was no specific information found on acute overdose in horses.

Drug Interactions

- Sucralfate and some antacids may interfere with the absorption of enrofloxacin. Dosing should be separated by at least two hours.
- Enrofloxacin may be used with aminoglycosides, some cephalosporins, and some penicillins in infections where it is warranted based on bacterial sensitivity.
- Enrofloxacin should not be used with chloramphenicol or rifampin.
- Enrofloxacin interferes with the metabolism of the bronchodilators, theophylline and aminophylline. If these drugs are to be used at the same time, blood levels should be monitored.

Special Considerations

- Enrofloxacin is well absorbed orally and intravenously. It is generally not used intramuscularly because it is too irritating.
- Enrofloxacin tastes terrible and some horses experience almost immediate oral mucous membrane irritation from this drug. Many veterinarians recommend diluting the drug with the sweetening agent of choice. The author has used enrofloxacin mixed with concentrated jello which was allowed to partially set up, similar to a "jello shot." It still tastes terrible but it syringes into their mouth well and does not cause irritation.
- Enrofloxacin is not FDA approved in the horse. It is commonly used and considered accepted practice. It is a prescription drug and U.S. federal law restricts this drug to use by or on the lawful written or oral order of a licensed veterinarian within the context of a valid veterinarian-client-patient relationship.

Special Populations

Breeding Animals

Enrofloxacin may cause articular cartilage abnormalities in young animals; consequently, many veterinarians are hesitant to use enrofloxacin in pregnant mares unless the benefits of therapy clearly outweigh the risks.

Foals

Because of the problems with cartilage abnormalities in young animals, enrofloxacin is not recommended for use in foals unless the benefits of therapy clearly outweigh the risks. If one is forced to use enrofloxacin in a young foal because of bacterial susceptibility, exercise should be severely restricted.

Ponies

Pony breeds do not appear to differ from horse breeds in their response to enrofloxacin.

Geriatrics

Enrofloxacin should be safe in older horses if liver and kidney functions are normal.

Competition Horses

Enrofloxacin is forbidden in any drug-free competition, but many regulatory groups do not prohibit antibiotics. Enrofloxacin is not restricted for horses showing under USEF's therapeutic substance rules. It is important to check with the individual regulatory organization.

Dose and Route of Administration

Oral: 3.4 mg/lb or 7.5 mg/kg once a day

Injectable: 3.4 mg/lb or 7.5 mg/kg once a day

Dose Form: 50 mg/ml or 100 mg/ml injectable, which may be used orally

AT A GLANCE:

FLUNIXIN MEGLUMINE

GENERIC NAME
Flunixin meglumine

COMMON BRAND NAME
Banamine, Citation,
Equileve, Meflosyl Solution

DRUG TYPE
Nonsteroidal anti-inflammatory
drug

INDICATIONS
Pain relief, anti-inflam-
matory, fever reduction,
endotoxemia, inflamma-
tion of the eye

Basic Information

Flunixin meglumine is a nonsteroidal anti-inflammatory drug
(NSAID). It is a potent pain reliever, fever reducer, and anti-inflammatory.

Flunixin is frequently used in the treatment of colic and other gastrointestinal (GI) disease for pain relief and for protection from toxins due to certain bacterial infections (endotoxemia). It is commonly used as an anti-inflammatory in the treatment of many painful eye
conditions.

Flunixin and other NSAIDs are also frequently prescribed to
reduce or control fevers due to viral or bacterial infections. These
drugs only provide symptomatic relief by lowering the fever. They do
not treat the underlying infection, and they can mask the severity of
the problem if used without appropriate veterinary evaluation and
therapy. Flunixin can be used for arthritis, although there are other
NSAIDs that are more commonly prescribed for this purpose.

NSAIDs work by inhibiting the body's production of prostaglandins
and other chemicals that stimulate the body's inflammatory response.
Some of the actions of NSAIDs may vary, depending on the amount
of the dose. NSAIDs are quickly absorbed into the blood stream. Pain
relief and fever reduction usually start within one to two hours.

Flunixin can be given orally or injected intramuscularly (IM) or
intravenously (IV).

Side Effects, Precautions, and Overdose

• GI ulceration, especially of the stomach and large colon, is the most common side effect.

• Rare side effects include kidney damage and bleeding disorders.

• Flunixin may be given IM, but injection-site reactions, including localized pain, swelling, and muscle inflammation or damage sometimes occur.

• Allergic reactions are rare but have been reported.

• NSAIDs should be avoided or very carefully monitored in horses with liver disease, kidney disease, or GI problems.

• A single miscalculated dose is not likely to produce toxicity. Experimentally it has taken three to five times the normal dose over multiple days to produce toxicity.

Drug Interactions

• This drug should not be combined with other anti-inflammatory drugs that tend to cause GI ulcers, such as corticosteroids and other NSAIDs.

• This drug should be used with caution with aminoglycoside antibiotics such as gentamicin and amikacin, and oral anticoagulants such as warfarin and other coumarin derivatives.

Special Considerations

• Some veterinarians may use more than one NSAID in combination, for example, flunixin and phenylbutazone given together. This is sometimes called stacking. Although there is little experimental evidence to support this practice, the theory is that different NSAIDs may act differently on different body systems. Particular care needs to be taken in this situation to avoid additive toxicity.

• Some veterinarians think that flunixin is sufficiently powerful that it can mask colic pain, making the decision regarding surgery more difficult. Many other veterinarians do not agree with that opinion and routinely use flunixin as their first-line drug in the treatment of colic. It is important to keep accurate records of all medications used to treat a horse with colic, particularly if the animal is referred to an equine hospital for intensive care or surgery.

• GI side effects such as ulcers are more likely to occur with prolonged oral dosing.

• Kidney problems are more likely to occur in the dehydrated or debilitated horse.

• Side effects from NSAID use are more common with phenylbutazone than with flunixin.

• Flunixin is FDA approved in the horse, and it is a prescription drug. U.S. federal law restricts this drug to use by or on the lawful written or oral order of a licensed veterinarian within the context of a valid veterinarian-client-patient relationship.

Special Populations

Breeding Animals

Although the effects of flunixin during pregnancy have not been studied, it is commonly used after manual twin reduction in early pregnancy. It is also commonly used to treat colic in the pregnant mare. Flunixin should be used with caution in the pregnant or nursing mare. No adverse effect on sperm production has been reported.

Foals

Flunixin is frequently used in foals, but it should be used with particular caution to avoid GI ulceration and maintain kidney function. Premature foals, septicemic foals, foals with questionable kidney or liver function, and foals with diarrhea require careful monitoring. Drugs to protect the GI tract such as omeprazole, cimetidine, or sucralfate are frequently used with flunixin.

Ponies

Pony breeds may be more susceptible to side effects from NSAIDs than horses. When NSAIDs are used in ponies, they should be used with caution and at the lowest effective dose.

Geriatrics

Older horses and especially those with decreased kidney or liver function may be more at risk for side effects. When flunixin is used in older horses, it should be used carefully and at the lowest effective dose.

Competition Horses

Flunixin is either a regulated or prohibited substance in most sanctioned competitions. It is a prohibited class A medication under the new FEI rules. USEF has a lengthy discussion of flunixin and other NSAIDs in its drug rules. Flunixin may be detected in a blood sample for two to three days. With the more sensitive ELISA test, it may be detected in urine samples for at least 15 days. Many regulatory agencies have a permissible drug level threshold. It is important to check with the individual regulatory group.

Dose and Route of Administration

Oral: 0.1 to 0.5 mg/lb, once a day. Do not exceed five days. Flunixin is well absorbed orally.

Injectable: 0.1 to 0.5 mg/lb, twice a day, IM or IV. Do not exceed five days.

Dose Form:

Oral: 1,500 mg paste syringe: 250 mg or 500 mg packet of granules

Injectable: 50 mg/ml

AT A GLANCE:

FUROSEMIDE

GENERIC NAME
Furosemide

COMMON BRAND NAME
Salix (formerly Lasix),
Furoject

DRUG TYPE
Diuretic

INDICATIONS
Exercise-induced pul-
monary hemorrhage,
congestive heart failure,
pulmonary edema, edema,
and non-inflammatory
swelling

Basic Information

Furosemide is the most commonly used diuretic in the horse. Diuretics are drugs that increase urine production and, consequently, decrease the amount of fluid within tissues and organs of the body. Diuretics act upon the kidneys, causing increased excretion of both electrolytes and water.

Diuretics such as furosemide are used to treat many types of fluid retention and excessive swelling, including pulmonary edema, some allergic reactions, and congestive heart failure. Furosemide is a commonly used drug in racehorses because it is thought to prevent or diminish the severity of exercise-induced pulmonary hemorrhage (EIPH) or bleeding from the lungs. Furosemide use in racehorses and its role in EIPH are controversial and hotly debated topics among veterinarians.

Although furosemide may cause a transient increase in blood flow to the kidneys, it does not improve kidney function and is not recommended for the treatment of most kidney diseases. Potent diuretics such as furosemide should always be used with caution because they can cause dehydration and electrolyte imbalances. Diuretics do little to relieve fluid accumulation and edema caused by low blood protein or inflammatory conditions such as vasculitis and infection.

Furosemide is given by injection in the muscle (IM) or in the vein (IV).

Side Effects, Precautions, and Overdose

• The most common side effects are dehydration and loss of electrolytes, including potassium, sodium, chloride, calcium, and magnesium. Potassium loss in particular can result in a clinical problem.

• Furosemide should not be given to animals in kidney failure, those that are dehydrated, or those likely to become dehydrated. It should be used with extreme caution in animals with electrolyte abnormalities or liver disease.

• Furosemide is not generally used as the sole therapy for congestive heart failure but is combined with other supportive cardiac drugs.

• In other species furosemide may cause damage to hearing and balance.

• Overdose of furosemide may cause dehydration and electrolyte imbalances. Signs include increased or decreased thirst and urination, lethargy, increased heart rate, gastrointestinal distress, seizures, collapse, and coma. Chronic overdose may cause kidney damage.

Drug Interactions

• There is a greater risk of electrolyte abnormalities (low blood potassium and calcium) when furosemide is given with corticosteroids.

• The dose of aspirin may need to be reduced in animals given furosemide.

• Furosemide can change the response to a number of drugs used during general anesthesia. It is important to inform the surgeon of furosemide and other medications if the animal is referred to an equine hospital for surgery.

• Furosemide increases the risk of kidney and ear damage from aminoglycoside antibiotics. Combined use of furosemide and trimethoprim sulfa may cause a decrease in platelet count.

Special Considerations

• The use of furosemide for the treatment or prevention of EIPH is controversial. The underlying causes, true incidence, and severity of EIPH are not entirely understood. Research in this field may produce changes in our understanding and treatment of this problem in the near future.

• In those states that permit furosemide in racehorses, the dose and administration of the drug are usually highly regulated.

• Some regulatory groups prohibit furosemide due to the common belief that furosemide can be used to mask the detection of other illegal drugs. Furosemide does not affect blood levels of other drugs, and the urine-diluting effect of furosemide is relatively short-lived.

• Furosemide is FDA approved in the horse, and it is a prescription drug. U.S. federal law restricts this drug to use by or on the lawful written or oral order of a licensed veterinarian within the context of a valid veterinarian-client-patient relationship.

Special Populations

Breeding Animals

In other species furosemide use during pregnancy has been shown to cause fetal deformities. In studies of other species, the drug is found to be excreted in the milk. Furosemide should not be used during pregnancy and with extreme care during lactation. No information was found regarding the safety of furosemide use in breeding stallions, although it is sometimes recommended to reduce acute swelling due to trauma to the penis or scrotum.

Foals

Foals are more at risk for dehydration and electrolyte abnormalities. Furosemide should be used with extreme care in foals.

Ponies

Pony breeds do not appear to differ from horses in their response to furosemide.

Geriatrics

Furosemide is safe to use in older animals if kidney and liver functions are normal. If kidney and liver functions are not normal, furosemide should be avoided. Furosemide should not be used in animals with pituitary pars intermedia dysfunction.

Competition Horses

Furosemide is commonly used and highly regulated in the racehorse. Different racing commissions have different protocols and rules for furosemide use. Detection time in the urine varies from 36 to 72 hours. Some states have a threshold level for blood samples. It is very important to check with the individual state racing authority in order to comply with that state's rules.

Furosemide is prohibited in any drug-free competition. USEF has provisions in its rules for the therapeutic use of prohibited substances; furosemide is forbidden under both the no foreign substance and therapeutic substance rules. It is important to check with the individual regulatory group.

Dose and Route of Administration

Injectable: 0.5 to 1.0 mg/lb, IV or IM, twice a day. The "pre-race" dose for EIPH is usually less.

Dose Form: 50 mg/ml

AT A GLANCE:

GRISEOFULVIN

GENERIC NAME
Griseofulvin

COMMON BRAND NAME
Fulvicin

DRUG TYPE
Fungistatic antibiotic

INDICATIONS
Ringworm and other
fungal skin conditions

Basic Information

Griseofulvin is a fungistatic antibiotic that is effective against the fungi that cause ringworm. It is used to treat fungal skin infections in many different species. The scientific name for those fungi that cause skin disease is dermatophyte, and the skin infection is called dermatophytosis. *Trichophyton* and *Microsporum* are the most common causes of ringworm or dermatophytosis in horses. *Trichophyton equinum* causes the large majority of the cases.

Griseofulvin is not effective against any bacterial infections or fungi other than the dermatophytes. It is rapidly absorbed and concentrates in the skin, hair, and hooves. Griseofulvin works by disrupting fungal reproduction, so it is effective in protecting new skin or hair growth from infection. However, it will not clear infection from hair or skin cells that are already involved.

Unfortunately, the most effective dose for griseofulvin in horses has not been established, and the efficacy of the currently recommended dose is questionable. Griseofulvin is relatively expensive, especially when compared to antifungal shampoos and other topical treatments.

Dermatophytes thrive in warm, moist, dirty environments. They invade the superficial skin layers through minor skin abrasion, or trauma. Infection causes hair loss, scales and crusts in the hairless areas, and itching. The hairless areas are often circular and patchy, giving the infection the common name of ringworm. The lesions are most commonly localized on the upper body but sometimes become generalized. Although the fungus is unsightly, the infection will run its course and is not life-threatening. Topical treatments are the first line of treatment and often cure the infection. It is difficult to recommend systemic treatment with griseofulvin except in selected cases of animals with underlying immune problems, or particularly difficult or severe infections.

Side Effects, Precautions, and Overdose

• There are few reported side effects from griseofulvin use in horses. In small animals griseofulvin can cause gastrointestinal (GI) upset. In humans rashes, irritability, memory loss, dizziness, and visual disturbances have also been reported.

• Griseofulvin is metabolized by the liver and should not be used in horses with decreased liver function.

• In safety studies horses have been given very large doses without signs of toxicity.

Drug Interactions

• Griseofulvin may reduce the activity of oral anticoagulants such as warfarin.

Special Considerations

• Many different species, including dogs, cats, and humans, may get ringworm.

• Ringworm is highly contagious. Management, including isolation, hygiene, and topical treatment, is very important to prevent its spread.

• Recommended topical treatments include clipping, exposing the lesions to sunlight, bathing with antifungal shampoos, and applying antifungal ointments to the lesions. Topical treatments should continue even if the animal is put on griseofulvin.

• The dermatophyte fungi survive well for more than one year in the environment on tack, blankets, and grooming equipment. Infections are usually spread by these items. Tack and grooming materials should not be shared and should be disinfected regularly.

• Most cases of ringworm will clear up on their own in 60 to 90 days due to the animal's natural immune response. Young horses are particularly susceptible to ringworm, probably because their immune systems are immature and they have not built up specific immunity from previous exposure.

• Reinfection is a constant risk without scrupulous attention to disinfection and management.

• Griseofulvin is FDA approved in the horse, and it is a prescription drug. U.S. federal law restricts this drug to use by or on the lawful written or oral order of a licensed veterinarian within the context of a valid veterinarian-client-patient relationship.

Special Populations

Breeding Animals

Griseofulvin should not be used in pregnant mares or breeding stallions. It has been demonstrated to cause fetal malformations in other species, and may possibly affect sperm production.

Foals

It is unlikely that griseofulvin would be used in young foals. The manufacturer gives a dose for foals but does not indicate a specific age.

Ponies

Pony breeds do not appear to differ from horse breeds in their response to griseofulvin.

Geriatrics

Griseofulvin should be safe in older horses if liver function is normal.

Competition Horses

Young racehorses are one of the groups with the highest incidence of skin disease. Griseofulvin is prohibited in any drug-free competition. Individual regulatory groups may have permissible detection levels. USEF has provisions in its rules for the therapeutic use of prohibited substances; griseofulvin is permitted for horses showing under the therapeutic substance rules. It is important to check with the individual regulatory body.

Dose and Route of Administration

Oral: Because the dose for griseofulvin is not well established, there are many different recommendations. Some veterinarians give the medication once a day for 30 to 60 days, and others give a larger dose once a week. A common dose is 2.5 to 5 mg/lb once a day.

Dose Form: 15-gram packets containing 2.5 grams of griseofulvin

AT A GLANCE:

HUMAN CHORIONIC GONADOTROPIN

GENERIC NAME
Human chorionic gonadotropin, HCG

COMMON BRAND NAME
Chorulon

DRUG TYPE
Hormone

INDICATIONS
Induce ovulation in mares, test for retained testicle in geldings/stallions

Basic Information

Human chorionic gonadotropin, also called chorionic gonadotropin or HCG, is a hormone secreted by the human placenta. It is harvested from the urine of pregnant women. It mimics the effect of the pituitary hormones, especially luteinizing hormone (LH). HCG acts primarily on the ovaries in females and on the testes in males.

HCG is widely used by broodmare veterinarians to induce ovulation in mares. HCG will usually cause ovulation of a mature follicle within 36 to 48 hours. Ideally, this permits the mare to be bred at the optimal time for conception and, therefore, fewer times per breeding cycle. This makes HCG an important management tool for both the mare owner and the stallion owner.

HCG may also be used in the diagnosis of retained testicles, or cryptorchidism. When a horse with a retained testicle is given HCG, it causes a measurable rise in testosterone. This HCG challenge test is a logical first step in diagnosing a gelding with stallion-like behavior.

HCG is usually given intramuscularly (IM), although some products may be labeled for intravenous (IV) use. Consult with your veterinarian.

Side Effects, Precautions, and Overdose

• There are no common side effects reported from HCG use. Injection site reactions such as pain and swelling are infrequent. These reactions usually respond to hot compresses and nonsteroidal anti-inflammatory drugs (NSAIDs). Contact your veterinarian if you notice a reaction. Rare anaphylactic reactions have been reported.

• HCG should not be given in early pregnancy as it may cause embryonic death.

• Repeated use of HCG may cause antibody formation in the mare. There is some thought that mares with high antibodies may not respond as reliably to HCG.

• No information on effects of overdose was found.

Drug Interactions

• There was no information found on drug interactions.

Special Considerations

• HCG can only induce mature follicles to ovulate. Follicles that are small or regressing are less likely to ovulate.

• HCG is less reliable early in the breeding season when mares are in their seasonal transition.

• Deslorelin, brand name Ovuplant, is a different product also used to induce ovulation in mares.

• Most HCG preparations have a limited shelf life once they are reconstituted. This will be listed on the label.

• HCG is FDA approved for use in cows. It is commonly used in horses and is accepted practice. HCG is a prescription drug. U.S. federal law restricts this drug to use by or on the lawful written or oral order of a licensed veterinarian within the context of a valid veterinarian-client-patient relationship.

Special Populations

Breeding Animals

HCG is regularly used in broodmares for the management of their heat cycles. No adverse effects on nursing foals have been noted. HCG is occasionally used in stallions.

Foals

HCG is not used in foals.

Ponies

Pony breeds are similar to horses in their response to HCG.

Geriatrics

HCG is not commonly used in older horses. It may be used in older broodmares and in the diagnosis of stallion-like behavior in older geldings.

Competition Horses

There are no indications for HCG use in competition horses. HCG is forbidden in drug-free competitions but may not be regulated under many types of rules. Check with the individual regulatory group.

Dose and Route of Administration

Injectable: 2,000 to 3,000 IU, given IM or IV

Dose Form: Powder for injection to be reconstituted with sterile water at 500 IU/ml, 1,000 IU/ml, or 2,000 IU/ml

AT A GLANCE:

HYALURONIC ACID

GENERIC NAME
Hyaluronic acid, Sodium
hyaluronate, HA

COMMON BRAND NAME
Hylartin, Hyalovet,
Hycoat, Hyvisc, Legend

DRUG TYPE
Disease-modifying osteoarthritis
agent, cartilage protective agent

INDICATIONS
Non-infectious, degenera-
tive, and/or traumatic
arthritis

Basic Information

Hyaluronic acid (or sodium hyaluronate) is a naturally occurring component of all connective tissues, including cartilage and joint fluid. It is chemically identical in all animal species, which allows the use of purified hyaluronic acid (HA) from cattle in horses. HA may be injected into joints or administered systemically to treat both acute and chronic joint damage. HA has been widely used in the joints of horses since the 1970s. The intravenous preparation came on the market in 1993. HA injection into joints has recently gained acceptance in some aspects of human orthopedics. HA is also available as a topical wound dressing. It is chemically related to the glycosaminoglycans. (See Polysulfated glycosaminoglycans.)

Normal joints have pads of cartilage protecting the ends of the bones that form the joint and a surrounding capsule lined by a synovial membrane. This membrane is very active in maintaining healthy joint function. Among its functions is the production of the lubricating joint fluid that helps to reduce friction and wear on the joint surfaces. Proteoglycans, a group of organic chemicals composed of protein and carbohydrate molecules, make up a large percentage of the cartilage, joint fluid, and synovial membrane. Hyaluronic acid and glycosaminoglycans such as chondroitin and glucosamine are major proteoglycans. HA is manufactured by the synovial lining of the joint and by the chondrocytes (cells that manufacture cartilage). HA forms a thin coating on articular cartilage and is a component of joint fluid.

Joint injury starts a cycle of inflammation, cartilage damage, and poor quality joint fluid that ultimately leads to irreversible damage and degenerative joint disease. The mechanism of action for HA supplementation or injections is not as simple as just providing better quality joint fluid or cushioning. It appears to have a direct anti-inflammatory effect in the joint and may affect the metabolism of some circulating white blood cells when given intravenously. It is thought to enhance healing by supporting connective tissue when used topically on wounds and as an adjunct to some soft tissue surgery.

Veterinarians, researchers, and academics sometimes argue over the merits of high molecular weight versus low molecular weight HA products. Both types of products are available on the market, and they both have their supporters. The lower molecular weight products are frequently less expensive.

Side Effects, Precautions, and Overdose

• Occasionally joint injections of HA will cause an acute inflammatory reaction in the joint. In these cases it is important to differentiate between a drug reaction and an infected joint. As a precaution against infection, some veterinarians add antibiotics to the HA when injecting a joint.

• It is very important to pay close attention to sterile or aseptic technique when injecting joints. Do not use HA in infected joints.

• Intra-articular injection should be avoided when the skin has been recently disturbed, blistered, fired, or has other skin problems.

• Systemic adverse reactions have not been reported with either the intra-articular or the intravenous products.

• HA is a very safe drug. Experimental overdoses, at five times the recommended dose for six weeks, caused no adverse effect.

Drug Interactions

• No drug interactions were reported.

Special Considerations

• The single most helpful treatment for any injured joint is rest. However, the use of anti-arthritic agents that protect and promote repair of cartilage in joints may be very desirable, especially when combined with other means of controlling inflammation.

• Horses treated intra-articularly with HA can be given nonsteroidal anti-inflammatory drugs for a few days after the joint injection. The horses are usually rested or put in light work for a few days after injection. Different veterinarians have different programs.

• Excess joint fluid is usually drained or removed before intra-articular injection of HA.

• Intra-articular injection with HA is commonly prescribed after joint surgery.

• HA is sometimes combined with corticosteroids when injected into joints for the treatment of acute inflammation.

• Polysulfated glycosaminoglycans may be given systemically along with HA.

• HA is FDA approved in the horse, and it is a prescription drug. U.S. federal law restricts this drug to use by or on the lawful written or oral order of a licensed veterinarian within the context of a valid veterinarian-client-patient relationship.

Special Populations

Breeding Animals

Limited reproductive studies have been done. Although it is not likely that these products would cause problems in breeding animals, they have not been extensively tested for this purpose. Use with caution in pregnant or lactating mares and in breeding stallions.

Foals

There are no specific contraindications to using this product in young animals.

Ponies

Pony breeds do not appear to differ from horses in their response to HA.

Geriatrics

HA is considered safe in older horses.

Competition Horses

HA is commonly used in competition horses. It is forbidden during some drug-free competitions but is not regulated under many other types of rules. Systemic HA may not be used during FEI competition. USEF has provisions in its rules for the therapeutic use of prohibited substances; HA is permitted for horses showing under the therapeutic substance rules. It is important to check with the individual regulatory group.

Dose and Route of Administration

Injectable:

Intra-articular: 10 to 40 mg/joint, depending on joint size. May be repeated once a week for three treatments.

Intravenous: 40 mg. May be repeated once a week for three treatments.

Dose Form:

Intra-articular: 2 ml sterile single dose syringe or vial

Intravenous: 4 ml single dose vial

Topical: 6 ml single dose vial

AT A GLANCE:

HYDROXYZINE

GENERIC NAME
Hydroxyzine

COMMON BRAND NAME
Atarax, Vistaril

DRUG TYPE
Antihistamine

INDICATIONS
Hives, itchy skin, and
other allergic skin problems

Basic Information

Hydroxyzine hydrochloride is an oral antihistamine used to treat
hives and itchy or bumpy allergic skin reactions in horses. Histamine
is a substance that is released from some types of cells if they are
damaged. It causes contraction of smooth muscle cells, including
those in the respiratory tract and intestines. It lowers blood pressure
by causing dilation of blood vessels. It causes the inflammation and
itching typical of allergic reactions.

Antihistamines do not block the release of histamine. Instead,
they compete with histamine for uptake at the histamine receptors
on sensitive cells in the respiratory tract, intestines, blood vessels,
and the skin.

Antihistamines generally take 20 to 45 minutes to exert an
effect after oral administration. They act more rapidly if given
systemically in the muscle or vein. The intravenous route is more
likely to cause side effects and is not commonly used. If antihistamines alone are unable to control all of the allergic signs, they
may be used with corticosteroids, allowing use of a lower dose of
the corticosteroids.

Side Effects, Precautions, and Overdose

Sedation is the most common side effect of antihistamine use.
Less common side effects include excitement, fine tremors, whole
body tremors, and seizures.

Individuals may react differently to antihistamines. The dose of hydroxyzine should be tailored to the individual horse.

- Overdoses cause increased sedation and increased risk of the other side effects already mentioned.

Drug Interactions

- Hydroxyzine has an additive effect when combined with other central nervous system depressant drugs such as tranquilizers.

Special Considerations

- Hydroxyzine is not FDA approved for use in horses. It is commonly used and considered accepted practice to do so. U.S. federal law restricts this drug to use by or on the lawful written or oral order of a licensed veterinarian within the context of a valid veterinarian-client-patient relationship.

Special Populations

Breeding Animals

High doses of antihistamines can cause birth defects in laboratory animals. It is not known if this occurs in horses. It is not known if hydroxyzine is excreted in milk. Hydroxyzine should only be used in pregnant or lactating animals if the benefits outweigh the risks.

Foals

No information was found on hydroxyzine use in foals. Carefully consider the risks and benefits before use.

Ponies

Pony breeds do not appear to differ from horses in their response to hydroxyzine.

Geriatrics

There are no studies in older horses. Older humans are more sensitive to side effects from antihistamines. A lower dose of hydroxyzine may be indicated in older horses.

Competition Horses

Hydroxyzine is prohibited or regulated in most sanctioned competitions. It is a prohibited class A medication under the new FEI rules. Oral drugs are much more likely to have variable detection times. Long-term or repeated doses can also affect detection times. USEF has provisions in its rules for the therapeutic use of prohibited substances. It is important to consult the individual regulatory group.

Dose and Route of Administration

Oral: 0.25 to 0.5 mg/lb, twice a day

Dose Form: Tablets: 10 mg, 15 mg, 50 mg, and 100 mg

AT A GLANCE:

ISOXSUPRINE

GENERIC NAME
Isoxsuprine hydrochloride

COMMON BRAND NAME
Generics

DRUG TYPE
Vasodilator

INDICATIONS
Navicular disease, laminitis

Basic Information

Isoxsuprine is most frequently used in horses for the management of navicular disease and laminitis although it is not a universally accepted treatment. Some veterinarians believe it helps, and others remain skeptical. This is partly because there has been conflicting research on the effects of isoxsuprine and partly because the underlying causes of navicular disease and laminitis are not completely understood.

Isoxsuprine is a vasodilator; it works by relaxing the smooth muscle around peripheral blood vessels. Impaired circulation and blood flow are probably contributing causes of both navicular disease and laminitis. Circulatory changes in the foot during laminitis are currently an area of intense research. As these diseases become better understood, improved methods of prevention and treatment are likely to evolve.

Side Effects, Precautions, and Overdose

• Side effects after oral administration are rare in the horse but can include changes in blood pressure, increased heart rate, and possible gastrointestinal irritation. In humans dizziness, weakness, and other central nervous system signs are also reported.

• Isoxsuprine is a vasodilator and should not be used in mares immediately after foaling or horses that are actively bleeding.

• Overdose of isoxsuprine increases the risk and severity of the aforementioned side effects.

Drug Interactions

• Isoxsuprine should be used with caution with other drugs that might affect blood pressure. That includes most sedatives and drugs used for general anesthesia. It is important to keep accurate records of isoxsuprine and any other medications used if an animal is referred to an equine hospital for intensive care or surgery.

Special Considerations

• In humans isoxsuprine is sometimes used in the treatment and management of premature labor. Some veterinarians have used isoxsuprine for the same purpose in broodmares, but its efficacy has not been scientifically established.

• Isoxsuprine is not FDA approved in the horse. It is commonly used and an accepted practice, and it is a prescription drug. U.S. federal law restricts this drug to use by or on the lawful written or oral order of a licensed veterinarian within the context of a valid veterinarian-client-patient relationship.

Special Populations

Breeding Animals

There are no safety studies on isoxsuprine use in pregnant or lactating mares. There are no safety studies on effects on semen in breeding stallions.

Foals

It is unlikely that isoxsuprine would be used in foals, and no information was found on this use.

Ponies

Pony breeds do not appear to differ from horses in their response to isoxsuprine.

Geriatrics

No information was found on isoxsuprine use in older horses. Isoxsuprine is metabolized by the liver. Liver function should be checked before administering isoxsuprine.

Competition Horses

Isoxsuprine is prohibited in any drug-free competition. It is permitted in some types of USEF competition and not in others. It is a prohibited class B medication under the new FEI rules. Oral drugs are much more likely to have variable detection times, and long-term or repeated doses can also affect detection times for many drugs. Detection time for isoxsuprine in urine is several weeks to months if the more sensitive ELISA test is used. It is important to consult with a knowledgeable veterinarian and the individual regulatory group.

Dose and Route of Administration

Oral: 0.1 to 0.3 mg/lb starting twice a day. This may be decreased to once a day. There are other dosing regimens.

Dose Form: 20 mg tablets

AT A GLANCE:

KETOPROFEN

GENERIC NAME
Ketoprofen

COMMON BRAND NAME
Ketofen

DRUG TYPE
Nonsteroidal anti-inflammatory drug

INDICATIONS
Pain relief especially for musculoskeletal pain, fever reduction, anti-inflammatory, endotoxemia

Basic Information

Ketoprofen is a nonsteroidal anti-inflammatory drug (NSAID). It is a potent pain reliever, fever reducer, and anti-inflammatory. Ketoprofen is frequently prescribed for musculoskeletal pain from soft tissue injury, bone and joint problems, or laminitis.

NSAIDs are used for musculoskeletal pain because they both relieve pain and decrease inflammation. They do not speed healing or cure the underlying problem, but they can make the horse more comfortable while he is recovering. Ketoprofen and other NSAIDs are also prescribed to reduce or control fevers due to viral or bacterial infections. These drugs only provide symptomatic relief by lowering the fever. They do not treat the underlying infection, and they can mask the severity of the problem if used without appropriate veterinary evaluation and therapy. Ketoprofen may also be used in the management of colic for protection from bacterial toxins (endotoxemia).

NSAIDs work by inhibiting the body's production of prostaglandins and other chemicals that stimulate the body's inflammatory response. Some of their actions may vary, depending on the amount of the dose. NSAIDs are quickly absorbed into the blood stream. Pain relief and fever reduction usually start within one to two hours.

Ketoprofen is only labeled for short-term use. The package insert recommends a maximum of five days. It is labeled for intravenous (IV) use only.

Side Effects, Precautions, and Overdose

• Side effects are uncommon when used at the recommended dose. The most common side effect includes ulceration of the gastrointestinal (GI) tract and a drop in the red blood cell count due to GI bleeding.

• Rare side effects include kidney damage, bleeding disorders, and protein loss.

• Ketoprofen is less likely to cause side effects than either flunixin or phenylbutazone.

• Injection site reactions can occur if blood or drug leaks back at the injection site.

• It should not be used in horses known to be allergic to aspirin.

• NSAIDs should be avoided or very carefully monitored in horses with liver disease, kidney disease, or GI problems.

• Overdoses of ketoprofen can cause GI ulcers, protein loss, and kidney and liver damage. Early signs of toxicity include loss of appetite and depression.

Drug Interactions

• Ketoprofen should not be combined with other anti-inflammatory drugs that tend to cause GI ulcers, such as corticosteroids and other NSAIDs.

• Ketoprofen should not be combined with anticoagulant drugs, particularly coumarin derivatives such as warfarin.

Special Considerations

• Some veterinarians may use more than one NSAID in combination, for example, ketoprofen and phenylbutazone given together. This is sometimes called stacking. Although there is little experimental evidence to support this practice, the theory is that different NSAIDs may act differently on different body systems. Particular care needs to be taken in this situation to avoid additive toxicity.

• Ketoprofen is not labeled for intramuscular use. Some veterinarians report using it in the muscle with only occasional injection site reactions.

• Ketoprofen is FDA approved in the horse, and it is a prescription drug. U.S. federal law restricts this drug to use by or on the lawful written or oral order of a licensed veterinarian within the context of a valid veterinarian-client-patient relationship.

Special Populations

Breeding Animals

Studies in other species showed no harmful effects in pregnant animals when used at normal doses. These studies have not been repeated in the horse, and the manufacturer cautions against ketoprofen's use in breeding animals. It is not known if it is present in the milk of horses. No adverse effects on sperm production have been reported in other species. Ketoprofen should only be used in breeding animals with caution, when the potential benefits outweigh the potential risks.

Foals

Ketoprofen may be used in foals, but it should be used with particular caution to avoid GI ulceration and maintain kidney function. Premature foals, septicemic foals, foals with questionable kidney or liver function, and foals with diarrhea require careful monitoring. Drugs to protect the GI tract such as omeprazole, cimetidine, and sucralfate are frequently used with NSAIDs.

Ponies

Pony breeds may be more susceptible to side effects from NSAIDs than horses. When NSAIDs are used in ponies, the drugs should be used with caution and at the lowest effective dose.

Geriatrics

Older horses, especially those with decreased kidney or liver function, may be more at risk for side effects. When ketoprofen is used in older horses, it should be used carefully and at the lowest effective dose.

Competition Horses

Ketoprofen is either a regulated or prohibited substance in most sanctioned competitions. It is a prohibited class A medication under the new FEI rules. USEF has a lengthy discussion of ketoprofen and other NSAIDs in its drug rules. Ketoprofen may be detected in blood or urine samples for up to five days. Urine samples are likely to test positive for longer than blood samples. Some regulatory groups may have a permissible detection level. It is important to consult with the individual regulatory group.

Dose and Route of Administration

Injectable: 1 mg/lb, IV, once a day

Dose Form: injectable 100 mg/ml

AT A GLANCE:

MACROLIDE ANTIBIOTICS

GENERIC NAME	COMMON BRAND NAME
Erythromycin	Ery-Tab, Robimycin, E-Mycin
Clarithromycin	Biaxin
Azithromycin	Zithromax

DRUG TYPE	INDICATIONS
Antibiotic	*Rhodococcus equi* (*R.equi*) infections

Basic Information

Erythromycin was the first macrolide antibiotic. It was isolated from soil bacteria in the early 1950s. Clarithromycin and azithromycin are newer semi-synthetic relatives of erythromycin. These drugs work by inhibiting the production of protein by susceptible bacteria. Therefore, they are usually bacteriostatic antibiotics. This family of antibiotics is most commonly used in foals for the treatment of disease caused by the bacteria *Rhodococcus equi*. They may be used alone or in combination with the antibiotic, rifampin.

R. equi pneumonia is the most severe, bacterial pneumonia in foals. Although *R. equi* usually causes respiratory disease, other systems can also be infected resulting in gastrointestinal (GI) abcessation and septic joints or septic growth plates. All forms of *R. equi* infection can be very difficult to diagnose and to treat because this bacterium tends to cause abscesses, and most antibiotics do not penetrate the abscesses in a high enough concentration to be effective. Fatalities can occur even with prompt diagnosis and treatment.

For many years, erythromycin, or erythromycin combined with rifampin, was the standard of care in the treatment of *R. equi* infections. Recently the two newer semi-synthetic macrolides have gained popularity in the treatment of this difficult disease. Azithromycin has better absorption characteristics than erythromycin. It concentrates in the cells in the lungs and in white blood cells. Azithromycin is a once-a-day drug and it may be less likely to cause GI problems. Clarithromycin is possibly the most effective drug of the three macrolide antibiotics for the treatment of *R. equi*. But there may be an increased incidence of diarrhea with this drug. Both azithromycin and clarithromycin are relatively expensive.

Side Effects, Precautions, and Overdose

• Side effects in foals for all three drugs include mild to moderate diarrhea and hyperthermia (heat-related illness) and increased body temperature. These side effects are potentially fatal. There is ample clinical evidence that foals on erythromycin are very sensitive to heat and possibly to bright sunlight. There have also been anecdotal reports of similar hyperthermia with both azithromycin and clarithromycin.

• Erythromycin is generally not used in horses one year of age or older. Severe, potentially fatal diarrhea can occur in these animals.

• Overdose of any macrolide antibiotic can cause severe GI side effects.

Drug Interactions

• Erythromycin, azithromycin, and clarithromycin may be combined with rifampin.

• Erythromycin is generally not used with chloramphenicol or penicillin antibiotics and should not be used with gentamicin.

• Erythromycin can delay clearance of the bronchodilator theophylline to the point of potential toxicity.

• Clarithromycin and omeprazole may increase the serum concentration of one another.

Special Considerations

• Most *R. equi* infections occur in hot, dry weather, making the management of the side effect of hyperthermia difficult. Because of this problem, many veterinarians do not turn foals on macrolide antibiotics out in the daytime and may severely limit their turnout time in general. Signs of hyperthermia include increased body temperature, panting, and respiratory distress. Aggressive cooling using cool water and fans or air conditioning is helpful.

• Foals being treated for *R. equi* may be on long-term antibiotics. The choice between the macrolide antibiotics will need to be made based on clinical response, ease or frequency of administration, and expense. Some foals tolerate one of these antibiotics better than another one.

• Oral erythromycin comes in a number of different chemical forms or "salts." They include erythromycin phosphate, stearate, estolate, or ethysuccinate. The dose and dosing frequency may vary with the form of the antibiotic used.

• Some veterinarians use oral probiotics in foals being treated with macrolide antibiotics in an attempt to decrease the likelihood or severity of antibiotic-induced diarrhea.

• Erythromycin is occasionally used intravenously in adult horses at a very low dose to improve intestinal motility as a part of medical management of colic.

• Erythromycin, clarithromycin, and azithromycin are not FDA approved in the horse. They are commonly used in foals and it is accepted practice. They are prescription drugs, and U.S. federal law restricts the use of these drugs by or on the lawful written or oral order of a licensed veterinarian within the context of a valid veterinarian-client-patient relationship.

Special Populations
Breeding Animals

Macrolide antibiotics are rarely used in adult horses. Although very rare, serious and potentially fatal diarrhea has been reported in mares whose suckling foals are on erythromycin. Extra care should be used to minimize or prevent any exposure to the mare. The water buckets and the foal's skin are common sources of exposure.

Foals

Macrolide antibiotics are almost exclusively used for the treatment of *R. equi* in foals.

Ponies

The indications for macrolide antibiotics use in pony foals are the same as in horse foals. Erythromycin is rarely used in adult ponies.

Geriatrics

Macrolide antibiotics are rarely used in adult horses.

Competition Horses

Macrolide antibiotics are rarely used in adult horses.

Dose and Route of Administration

Erythromycin

Oral: 11-14 mg/lb, three or four times a day

Dose Form: 250 mg and 500 mg tablets.

Azithromycin

Oral: 4.5 mg/lb or 10 mg/kg, once a day for 5-7 days, then every other day

Dose Form: Usually the human product is compounded into a paste form.

Clarithromycin

Oral: 3.4 mg/lb or 7.5 mg/kg, twice a day

Dose Form: Usually the human product is compounded into a paste form.

AT A GLANCE:

MECLOFENAMIC ACID

GENERIC NAME
Meclofenamic acid

COMMON BRAND NAME
Arquel

DRUG TYPE
Nonsteroidal anti-inflammatory
drug

INDICATIONS
Pain relief, particularly
for musculoskeletal pain,
anti-inflammatory, fever
reduction

Basic Information

Meclofenamic acid is a nonsteroidal anti-inflammatory drug (NSAID). All NSAIDs relieve pain and reduce fever. The pharmacological effects of this drug are similar to those of aspirin. It is frequently prescribed for musculoskeletal pain from soft tissue injury, bone and joint problems, and occasionally laminitis.

NSAIDs work by inhibiting the body's production of prostaglandins and other chemicals that stimulate the body's inflammatory response. They do not speed healing or cure the underlying problem, but they can make the horse more comfortable while he is recovering. Meclofenamic acid is well absorbed after oral administration, but it may take a day or two before the effects are seen. Other NSAIDs are more commonly used for colic and for other acute problems such as reducing fevers.

Side Effects, Precautions, and Overdose

• Adverse reactions are uncommon. The most common side effects include ulceration of the mouth and gastrointestinal (GI) tract, GI bleeding, colic, and diarrhea. Decreased red blood cell count due to bleeding may occur.

• Horses with heavy bot infestations may be more likely to have GI problems.

- NSAIDs should be avoided or very carefully monitored in horses with active liver disease, kidney disease, or GI problems.
- Meclofenamic acid should be avoided in horses known to be allergic to aspirin.
- Early signs of toxicity include loss of appetite, colic, diarrhea, ulcers in the mouth, and depression.

Drug Interactions
- Avoid combining meclofenamic acid with other anti-inflammatory drugs that tend to cause GI ulcers, such as corticosteroids and other NSAIDs. In particular, combining with aspirin may increase blood loss due to GI side effects.
- Avoid combining meclofenamic acid with anticoagulant drugs such as warfarin and other coumarin derivatives and sulfa antibiotics.

Special Considerations
- Some veterinarians may use more than one NSAID in combination. This is sometimes called stacking. Although there is little experimental evidence to support this practice, the theory is that different NSAIDs may act differently on different body systems. Particular care needs to be taken in this situation to avoid potential toxicity.
- Meclofenamic acid is FDA approved in the horse, and it is a prescription drug. U.S. federal law restricts this drug to use by or on the lawful written or oral order of a licensed veterinarian within the context of a valid veterinarian-client-patient relationship.

Special Populations
Breeding Animals
Studies in other animals have shown that meclofenamic acid can delay labor and cause skeletal abnormalities in the fetus. It can cross the placenta and is found in milk. Although these effects have not been shown in the horse, meclofenamic acid should only be used in the pregnant or nursing mare when the potential benefits are care-

fully weighed against the possible risks. No adverse effect on sperm production has been reported.

Foals

Meclofenamic acid is not commonly used in foals. If used, it should be used with particular caution to avoid GI ulceration and maintain kidney function. Premature foals, septicemic foals, foals with questionable kidney or liver function, and foals with diarrhea require careful monitoring. Drugs to protect the GI tract such as omeprazole, cimetidine, and sucralfate are frequently used with meclofenamic acid.

Ponies

Pony breeds may be more susceptible to side effects from NSAIDs than horses. When NSAIDs are used in ponies, the drugs should be used with caution and at the lowest effective dose.

Geriatrics

Older horses, especially those with decreased kidney or liver function, may be more susceptible to side effects from NSAIDs. When these drugs are used in an older horse, they should be used at the lowest effective dose.

Competition Horses

Meclofenamic acid is either a regulated or prohibited substance in most sanctioned competitions. It is a prohibited class A medication under the new FEI rules. USEF has a lengthy discussion of NSAIDs, including meclofenamic acid, in its drug rules. Meclofenamic acid may be detected in blood or urine samples for two to four days, depending on the sensitivity of the test. Many regulatory agencies have a permissible drug level threshold. It is important to check with the individual regulatory group.

Dose and Route of Administration

Oral: 1 mg/lb once a day for five to seven days then decrease the dose and increase the interval to obtain the lowest effective dose

Dose Form: 10 gram packets containing 500 mg meclofenamic acid

AT A GLANCE:

METHOCARBAMOL

GENERIC NAME
Methocarbamol

COMMON BRAND NAME
Robaxin

DRUG TYPE
Muscle relaxant

INDICATIONS
Reduction of muscle
spasm due to trauma or
inflammation

Basic Information

Methocarbamol is a centrally acting muscle relaxant. Interestingly, it does not work on skeletal muscle directly, but instead works on the central nervous system (CNS).

Methocarbamol is used to treat muscle spasms associated with back problems and exercise-related muscle problems such as tying up. It may also be used as part of the treatment for tetanus. Methocarbamol is safe to use with nonsteroidal anti-inflammatory drugs, corticosteroids, and other medications used for the treatment of muscle spasm.

Side Effects, Precautions, and Overdose

• The most common side effect is sedation.

• Methocarbamol is a CNS depressant. At normal doses it is considered a safe and relatively nontoxic drug. Salivation and staggering are sometimes seen after rapid intravenous (IV) administration.

• Injectable methocarbamol contains polyethylene glycol and should probably not be used in animals with decreased kidney function. Particular care should be used when giving methocarbamol to horses that are dehydrated or with severe symptoms of tying up. In horses that are severely tied up, especially those with discolored urine, simultaneous treatment with large volumes of intravenous fluids is frequently recommended.

• Because methocarbamol can cause sedation and CNS depression, it may impair coordination.

- Injection site reactions can occur if blood leaks back at the injection site.
- Overdoses usually cause CNS depression, excessive sedation, staggering, altered reflexes, and prostration.

Drug Interactions

- Methocarbamol will cause additive CNS depression if given with other drugs that depress the central nervous system.

Special Considerations

- Oral methocarbamol is sometimes prescribed for preventative use in horses that are prone to tying up.
- Injectable methocarbamol is FDA approved in the horse. Oral methocarbamol is a human drug and is not FDA approved in the horse. However, it is commonly used and is accepted practice. Methocarbamol is a prescription drug. U.S. federal law restricts this drug to use by or on the lawful written or oral order of a licensed veterinarian within the context of a valid veterinarian-client-patient relationship.

Special Populations

Breeding Animals

Studies in the rat show no harmful effects from methocarbamol in the pregnant rat or fetus. No other animal studies have been performed. It is not known if methocarbamol is excreted in milk. There is no information regarding safety in breeding stallions. The lack of information should encourage caution with careful consideration of risks and benefits before using methocarbamol in breeding animals.

Foals

There is no information regarding safety in foals. Methocarbamol is used in children with tetanus. Again, consider potential risks and benefits before using in foals.

Ponies

There are no contraindications for use in ponies.

Geriatrics

There are no contraindications for use in older horses with normal kidney function.

Competition Horses

Methocarbamol is either a regulated or prohibited substance in most sanctioned competitions. It is a prohibited class A medication under the new FEI rules. It may be detected in the blood for approximately 72 hours. Detection times may depend on the amount given and may vary further with oral use. Some regulatory agencies have a permissible drug level threshold. USEF has issued general recommendations concerning doses and times to help competitors comply with its restrictions. It is important to check with the individual regulatory organization.

Dose and Route of Administration

Oral: 2 to 5 mg/lb, twice a day

Injectable: 2 to 25 mg/lb, four times a day, IV only. The higher dose range is used in the treatment of tetanus.

Dose Form:

Injectable: 100 mg/ml

Oral tablets for humans: 500 mg and 750 mg

AT A GLANCE:

METRONIDAZOLE

GENERIC NAME
Metronidazole

COMMON BRAND NAME
Flagyl, Protostat

DRUG TYPE
Antibiotic, antiprotozoal

INDICATIONS
Anaerobic bacterial infections, Giardia

Basic Information

Metronidazole is primarily used as an antibiotic to treat anaerobic bacterial infections. These are bacteria that cannot live in the presence of oxygen as opposed to aerobic bacteria that require oxygen to live. Metronidazole may also be used as an antiprotozoal to treat Giardia infections. (Giardia causes an infectious form of diarrhea.) It kills susceptible organisms by disrupting their DNA. Metronidazole is rapidly absorbed from the gastrointestinal tract into the blood stream.

Metronidazole is used with other antibiotics to treat bacterial infections that cause pleuropneumonia, peritonitis, abdominal abscesses, and other severe infections caused by a mixture of aerobic and anaerobic bacteria. It is also prescribed to prevent infection after colic or other abdominal surgery when mixed bacterial infections are a risk.

Side Effects, Precautions, and Overdose

- Side effects are not commonly associated with metronidazole. The major problem with using this drug in animals is its bad taste. Many horses stop eating when this drug is mixed with feed, and a reliable method of administration must be found.

- In other species of animals, neurologic signs are sometimes observed when an animal is on long-term, moderate-to-high doses.

• No information was found on overdose in the horse. In other species, loss of appetite, depression, and neurologic signs are reported.

Drug Interactions

• Metronidazole increases the effect of anticoagulants such as warfarin.

• Cimetidine can interfere with the liver's ability to break down metronidazole, and the dose may have to be reduced.

Special Considerations

• The types of mixed bacterial infections where metronidazole is commonly used are difficult to cure and frequently require long-term administration of antibiotics.

• Metronidazole is absorbed rectally. This route can be used in the very sick patient when weight loss and appetite loss are problems.

• Metronidazole is not FDA approved for use in horses, but it is commonly used and considered accepted practice to do so. U.S. federal law restricts this drug to use by or on the lawful written or oral order of a licensed veterinarian within the context of a valid veterinarian-client-patient relationship.

Special Populations

Breeding Animals

Metronidazole causes birth defects in laboratory animals. It should be avoided in pregnant animals, especially in the first trimester. Some metronidazole is excreted in breast milk, and it should not be used in lactating animals. There is no information available on the safety of metronidazole in breeding stallions.

Foals

There are no specific contraindications to metronidazole use in foals.

Ponies

There are no specific contraindications to metronidazole use in ponies.

Geriatrics

Metronidazole is safe to use in older animals if liver function is normal. If liver function is not normal, metronidazole should be avoided or the dose should be decreased.

Competition Horses

Metronidazole would be forbidden in any drug-free competition, but many regulatory groups do not prohibit antibiotics. Antibiotics are not restricted for horses showing under the therapeutic substance rules of USEF. It is important to check with the individual regulatory organization.

Dose and Route of Administration

Oral: 7 to 11 mg/lb, two to four times a day

Dose Form: 250 mg, 375 mg, and 500 mg capsules or tablets

AT A GLANCE:

N-BUTYLSCOPOLAMMONIUM BROMIDE

GENERIC NAME
N-butylscopolammonium bromide

COMMON BRAND NAME
Buscopan

DRUG TYPE
Antispasmodic and anticholinergic

INDICATIONS
Spasmodic or gas colic, rectal examination

Basic Information

N-butylscopolammonium bromide is a drug that has been used for many years in Europe as a first line of treatment for minor gas colic. N-butylscopolammonium bromide is a short-acting antispasmodic with no sedative properties; therefore, it is unlikely to mask a more serious medical or surgical emergency. It has a short duration of action of about 30 minutes. With proper case selection, this makes it an attractive drug for the early treatment of gas colic.

As might be expected from a drug that causes smooth muscle relaxation, N-butylscopolammonium bromide has been found to be effective in causing rectal relaxation and decreasing rectal straining. This makes it a useful drug for patients in which straining makes rectal examination difficult or risky for the patient. Some practitioners also use N-butylscopolammonium bromide to cause smooth muscle relaxation of the esophagus when treating a case of esophageal obstruction or "choke."

Side Effects, Precautions, and Overdose

• N-butylscopolammonium bromide should not be used in abdominal pain where ileus (lack of gastrointestinal activity) is a component.

• Although N-butylscopolammonium bromide is labeled for impaction colic, case selection will be important as some impactions are prone to ileus.

- N-butylscopolammonium bromide will cause a temporary increase in heart rate for about 30 minutes. It may also cause temporary dilation of the pupils.
- Safety studies were conducted at up to 10 times the recommended dose. Overdose of N-butylscopolammonium bromide caused an increase in duration and severity of side effects, and some mild colic.

Drug Interactions
- The effects of N-butylscopolammonium bromide may be increased when used with other anticholinergic drugs.

Special Considerations
- Veterinarians frequently use heart rate as a partial indicator of severity of pain. Because N-butylscopolammonium bromide causes a transient increase in heart rate, one would need to wait for approximately 30 minutes in order to use heart rate as a part of the clinical picture.
- In Europe, this drug is sold as a combination product with dipyrone. The dipyrone component provides pain relief in addition to the smooth muscle relaxation provided by the N-butylscopolammonium bromide.

Special Populations
Breeding Animals
The safety of this drug has not been established in pregnant or lactating mares.

Foals
The safety of this drug has not been established in foals.

Ponies
Pony breeds are similar to horses in their response to this drug.

Geriatrics

There is no additional information regarding older horses and the use of this drug.

Competition Horses

N-butylscopolammonium bromide is a prohibited substance in most sanctioned competitions. It is a prohibited class B drug under the new FEI rules. It may be used during USEF competitions under the therapeutic substance rule by observing a 24-hour withdrawal period and filling out the proper paperwork. Detection time varies but is in the range of seven days. It is important to check with the individual regulatory group.

Dose and Route of Administration

Injectable: 0.14 mg/lb or 0.3 mg/kg by slow intravenous injection
Dose Form: 20 mg/ml injectable

AT A GLANCE:

NAPROXEN

GENERIC NAME
Naproxen

COMMON BRAND NAME
Naprosyn

DRUG TYPE
Nonsteroidal anti-inflammatory
drug

INDICATIONS
Pain relief, particularly
for musculoskeletal pain,
anti-inflammatory

Basic Information

Naproxen is a nonsteroidal anti-inflammatory drug (NSAID) and a potent pain reliever. Naproxen is prescribed for lameness, musculoskeletal pain from soft tissue injury, muscle soreness, and bone and joint problems.

NSAIDs are used for musculoskeletal pain because they both relieve pain and decrease inflammation. They do not speed healing or cure the underlying problem, but they can make the horse more comfortable while recovering. They work by inhibiting the body's production of prostaglandins and other chemicals that stimulate the body's inflammatory response.

Different NSAID drugs are used to treat different medical problems. For example, naproxen is generally used for musculoskeletal problems whereas flunixin is more commonly used for pain relief for colic. Although NSAIDs are quickly absorbed into the blood stream, response time can vary greatly among different NSAIDs. Naproxen is absorbed promptly, but full clinical response may not occur for five to seven days. Meclofenamic acid may take two to three days for full clinical response, but flunixin can provide relief for colic pain in less than an hour. Some of the actions of NSAID drugs may vary, depending on the amount of the dose.

Side Effects, Precautions, and Overdose

• Adverse reactions to naproxen are uncommon in the horse. The most common side effects are gastrointestinal (GI) problems such as ulcers, diarrhea, and GI pain.

• Rare side effects include kidney damage, bleeding disorders, and protein loss.

• NSAIDs should be avoided or very carefully monitored in horses with liver disease, kidney disease, or GI problems.

• Overdoses of naproxen cause more severe manifestations of the side effects. Early signs of toxicity include loss of appetite, colic, and depression.

Drug Interactions

• Naproxen should not be combined with other anti-inflammatory drugs that tend to cause GI ulcers, such as corticosteroids and other NSAIDs. In particular, the combination of naproxen with aspirin may increase blood loss due to GI side effects.

• Naproxen should not be combined with anticoagulant drugs such as warfarin and other coumarin derivatives, or sulfa antibiotics.

• Naproxen may decrease the diuretic activity of furosemide.

Special Considerations

• Some veterinarians may use more than one NSAID in combination. This is sometimes called stacking. Although there is little experimental evidence to support this practice, the theory is that different NSAIDs may act differently on different body systems. Particular care needs to be taken if this is done to avoid additive toxicity.

• Response to naproxen may not be apparent for five to seven days.

• Naproxen was once sold as a veterinary product under the brand name Equiproxen. It is now only available as a human product. It is a prescription drug. U.S. federal law restricts this drug to use by or on the lawful written or oral order of a licensed veterinarian within the context of a valid veterinarian-client-patient relationship.

Special Populations

Breeding Animals

Work in other animal species has shown no adverse effect from naproxen on pregnancy or fetal well being. This work has not been repeated in the horse. Naproxen should be used with caution in the pregnant or nursing mare and only when the benefits outweigh the risks. No adverse effect on sperm production has been reported.

Foals

Naproxen is not commonly used in foals. If it is used, it should be used with particular caution to avoid GI ulceration and maintain kidney function. Premature foals, septicemic foals, foals with questionable kidney or liver function, and foals with diarrhea require careful monitoring. Drugs to protect the GI tract such as omeprazole, cimetidine, and sucralfate are frequently used with naproxen.

Ponies

Pony breeds may be more susceptible to side effects from NSAIDs than horses. When NSAIDs are used in ponies, the drugs should be used with caution and at the lowest effective dose.

Geriatrics

Older horses, especially those with decreased kidney or liver function, may be more susceptible to side effects from NSAIDs. When these drugs are used in an older horse, they should be used at the lowest effective dose.

Competition Horses

Naproxen is either a regulated or prohibited substance in most sanctioned competitions. It is a prohibited class A medication under the new FEI rules. USEF has a lengthy discussion of NSAIDs, including naproxen, in its drug rules. Naproxen may be detected in urine samples for up to five days, depending on the sensitivity of the test.

Some regulatory agencies may have a permissible drug level threshold. It is important to check with the individual regulatory group.

Dose and Route of Administration

Oral: 4 mg/lb, once or twice a day for up to 14 days

Dose Form: 500 mg tablets

AT A GLANCE:

NITAZOXANIDE

GENERIC NAME
Nitazoxanide

COMMON BRAND NAME
Navigator

DRUG TYPE
Antiparasitic
Antiprotozoal

INDICATIONS
Equine protozoal
myeloencephalitis

Basic Information

Nitazoxanide is a drug with activity against a variety of parasites including protozoa, Giardia, nematodes, trematodes, and some bacteria. It is FDA approved for use in the horse to treat *Sarcocystis neurona*, the protozoa that cause equine protozoal myeloencephalitis (EPM). It is also used for the treatment of Giardia in humans, and there is considerable interest in this drug for use in other species.

Nitazoxanide is a "cidal" drug. Although the mechanism is not entirely understood, it is thought that it may kill the parasite by disrupting a stage of its energy metabolism. The course of treatment with nitazoxanide is 28 days long, which is based both on properties of the drug and the life cycle of the parasite.

The problem with all treatments for EPM is that the damage to the central nervous system caused by the protozoa parasite may be irreversible. After a successful course of treatment, the animal may no longer have EPM but may remain to some degree neurologically damaged. In the case of nitazoxanide, the manufacturer claims that in their larger field study, 81% of the treated animals improved, which again means better but not necessarily "normal." The degree of permanent damage is not entirely predictable, but as with any disease early diagnosis and treatment are more likely to produce a successful outcome. When evaluating this drug and others for effectiveness, it is important to give the animal enough time to stabilize and rehabilitate from the disease.

Side Effects, Precautions, and Overdose

• This is a tough drug on the patient because there is a relatively high incidence of side effects. Horses being treated with this drug should be under a veterinarian's care and monitored closely.

• Common side effects include decreased appetite, fever, depression, increased or decreased gut sounds, diarrhea or decreased manure production, colic, laminitis, discolored urine, increased water consumption, swelling of the head or legs, and weight loss.

• The most serious side effect is a potentially fatal drug-related diarrhea, or enterocolitis. This is due to disruption and change of the gastrointestinal bacteria. Horses on nitazoxanide should be watched closely for fever, colic, and diarrhea. A veterinarian will need to evaluate the horse at the first sign of trouble.

• Horses being treated with nitazoxanide may have what is referred to as a "treatment crisis" during the first two weeks of treatment. This may include worsening of the neurological signs, fever, decreased appetite, and lethargy. It is thought that the treatment crisis is precipitated by the killing of the parasite and inflammation in the central nervous system. These horses may need to be treated with anti-inflammatory drugs and will require additional close monitoring. Some horses may need to discontinue treatment.

• Nitazoxanide should be used with additional caution in animals with decreased liver or kidney function.

• It is very important to monitor the patient's weight in order to dose this drug accurately. There is a relatively narrow margin of safety.

• In safety studies performed by the manufacturer, a single overdose of five times the normal dose was given to eight horses. All of the horses developed side effects such as those described above but all of them survived.

Drug Interactions

• Information supplied by the manufacturer indicates that nitazoxanide has been used during the field studies with tranquilizers, antibiotics, nonsteroidal anti-inflammatory drugs, corticosteroids, wormers, diuretics, and vaccines without an increased incidence of adverse reaction. No specific drug interactions have been noted at this time.

Special Considerations

• There is a client information sheet that comes with nitazoxanide. The instructions are quite specific and should be followed closely.

• Adverse reactions are treated with a variety of drugs including NSAIDs, DMSO, dexamethasone, probiotics, antibiotics, oral electrolytes, and mineral oil.

• Animals receiving nitazoxanide should not be subjected to additional stress such as shipping or to abrupt changes in stabling, diet, or exercise routine.

• In field studies performed by the manufacturer, 27% to 31% of the treated horses experienced some form of adverse reaction, with a couple of fatalities occurring. The majority of the adverse reactions occurred within the first 10 days.

• Nitazoxanide is FDA approved in the horse, and it is a prescription drug. Federal law restricts this drug to use by or on the order of a licensed veterinarian.

Special Populations

Breeding Animals

Although the manufacturer does not make drug safety claims in the pregnant mare, in studies using nitazoxanide in pregnant mares there were no additional pregnancy-related problems. The manufacturer states: "Stallions may be more prone to develop laminitis while on this drug." Nitazoxanide should be used with caution in these populations and only when the benefits clearly outweigh the risk of treatment.

Foals

Foals do not commonly develop EPM. The manufacturer does not recommend nitazoxanide in animals less than one year old.

Ponies

The manufacturer recommends additional caution regarding the use of this drug in any group that may be more prone to developing laminitis. Because many pony breeds are prone to laminitis, nitazoxanide should only be used when the benefits clearly outweigh the risk of treatment.

Geriatrics

The manufacturer recommends additional caution regarding the use of this drug in any group that may be more prone to developing laminitis. Two common problems in older horses which make these horses more prone to laminitis are pituitary pars intermedia dysfunction and insulin resistance. Nitazoxanide should only be used in these horses when the benefits clearly outweigh the risk of treatment.

Competition Horses

It is unlikely that nitazoxanide would be used in horses that are competing. Should the circumstances arise, it would be important to consult with the individual regulatory group.

Dose and Route of Administration

Oral: 11.36 mg/lb orally once a day for five days followed by 22.72 mg/lb orally once a day

Dose Form: Calibrated paste syringe. Dispensing box contains 28-day course of treatment for a 1,200-lb horse.

AT A GLANCE:

OMEPRAZOLE

GENERIC NAME
Omeprazole

COMMON BRAND NAME
GastroGard, UlcerGard

DRUG TYPE
Gastric acid (proton) pump
inhibitor

INDICATIONS
Equine gastric ulcer
disease

Basic Information

Omeprazole is from a new class of drugs called gastric acid (proton) pump inhibitors. It is one of the anti-ulcer medications that prevent the secretion of acid in the stomach. These drugs stop the production of stomach acid by a mechanism that is different from cimetidine, ranitidine, and the other H_2 antagonists. Omeprazole is well absorbed after oral administration and metabolized primarily in the liver. It is effective both in treating the symptoms of ulcers and in preventing ulcers from occurring in those at risk.

Omeprazole is frequently an effective treatment of ulcers that are not responsive to the H_2 blockers or sucralfate. It is the only drug shown to resolve ulcers in horses in training without modification of the training schedule. This is very important, particularly for racing and performance horses.

Equine gastric ulcer disease (EGUD) is a complex disease. There are many contributing factors including age, use of the horse, diet, medications, stress, training, stabling conditions, weather conditions, and illness to name a few. Racehorses and foals are two populations at increased risk for gastric ulcers. More often than not, a combination of factors is involved in ulcer development. The location of the ulcers within the stomach and upper gastrointestinal tract can vary, and this influences which medications are likely to be effective. Our knowledge of the diagnosis and treatment of EGUD has exploded in the last 10 years primarily due to increased endoscopic examination of the stomach. Endoscopy has allowed accurate diagnosis as well as documenting the response to treatment.

Side Effects, Precautions, and Overdose

• Omeprazole is generally a very safe medication. No adverse side effects are listed in the manufacturer's package insert.

• Omeprazole should be used with caution in animals with liver disease or decreased liver function. The dosage may need to be decreased.

• Clinical experience with overdoses of omeprazole is very limited. There is a very wide margin of safety reported in safety trials done by the manufacturer.

Drug Interactions

• Omeprazole may affect the clearance of anticoagulants such as warfarin.

• The manufacturer states that omeprazole was used with a variety of commonly used equine medications, including dewormers, vaccines, antibiotics, diuretics, tranquilizers, nonsteroidal anti-inflammatories (NSAIDs), and corticosteroids without adverse drug interactions.

Special Considerations

• Omeprazole and other anti-ulcer drugs are sometimes prescribed as a precaution with NSAIDS, corticosteroids, and other drugs that can cause stomach ulcers.

• Maximum suppression of acid production occurs three to five days after the start of treatment.

• Omeprazole is FDA approved in the horse, and it is a prescription drug. U.S. federal law restricts this drug to use by or on the lawful written or oral order of a licensed veterinarian within the context of a valid veterinarian-client-patient relationship.

Special Populations

Breeding Animals

Omeprazole has not been studied in pregnant mares. It is unknown if omeprazole is excreted in milk. It should be avoided unless the benefits outweigh the potential risks. Small safety trials performed by the manufacturer on stallions showed no detrimental effect on semen quality or breeding behavior.

Foals

Omeprazole is frequently used in foals at risk for equine gastric ulcer disease.

Ponies

Pony breeds do not appear to differ from horses in their response to omeprazole.

Geriatrics

Omeprazole should be safe in older animals if liver function is adequate.

Competition Horses

Omeprazole is commonly used in competition horses, as these horses, as a population, appear to have a relatively higher incidence of EGUD. Individual racing commissions may have established permitted detection levels for this drug.

Omeprazole is permitted for horses showing under the therapeutic substance rules of USEF. The FEI also now permits the use of omeprazole during FEI competitions. It is important to check with a knowledgeable veterinarian and with the individual regulatory agency.

Dose and Route of Administration

Oral: Treatment of gastric ulcers: 1.8 mg/lb, once a day for four weeks

Prevention of recurrence of gastric ulcers: 0.9 mg/lb, once a day for four weeks

Dose Form: Paste syringe calibrated by weight. One syringe per day for 1,250-lb horse provides 1.8 mg/lb.

AT A GLANCE:

OXYTOCIN

GENERIC NAME
Oxytocin

COMMON BRAND NAME
Pitocin, Oxoject, generics

DRUG TYPE
Hormone

INDICATIONS
Stimulation of uterine contractions and milk letdown

Basic Information

Oxytocin is a hormone that is produced and stored in the brain. In females, oxytocin is released during labor, causing contractions of the uterus and milk letdown. A foal sucking also causes oxytocin release, which, in turn, causes milk letdown. Oxytocin does not directly stimulate the production of milk, only its ejection from the udder.

Oxytocin has many uses in the management of broodmares, both at the time of foaling and at the time of breeding. It is used to induce labor or to increase contractions during a difficult labor. After the mare foals, it may be used to stimulate contractions that help detach a retained placenta, to contract the uterus in order to control uterine bleeding, or to contract the uterus after the replacement of a uterine prolapse (when all or part of the uterus is expelled through the vulva). Recently oxytocin has become widely used to stimulate the evacuation of excess fluid from the uterus of mares after breeding or after uterine lavage.

Side Effects, Precautions, and Overdose

• The most common side effects to oxytocin are sweating, cramping, and colicky discomfort.

• Oxytocin should not be used when the fetus is in an abnormal position or is too large to pass through the birth canal.

• Inappropriate use of oxytocin, including overdose, can cause excessive uterine contractions and possible rupture.

Drug Interactions

• No drug interactions were found for the horse.

Special Considerations

• Induction of labor in mares is somewhat controversial. It is diffi-cult to predict fetal maturity based solely on the number of days of ges-tation. A number of guidelines for the mare's "readiness to deliver" have been published. They include a minimum number of days of ges-tation, softening of the cervix, presence of colostrum in the udder, and relaxation of the pelvic ligaments and vulva. Artificial induction of labor has significant risks of complication to both the mare and the foal. There are medical circumstances when the induction of labor is appropriate, but only after full consideration of the risks and benefits.

• Research has shown that some mares are more susceptible to uterine infections post-breeding because of delayed clearance of inflammatory fluids from the uterus. These mares frequently have an enlarged, pendulous uterus and retained fluid can be seen on ultra-sound examination. Low doses of oxytocin may be useful in the post-breeding management of these mares.

• Oxytocin can improve milk letdown, but it does not increase milk production. Lack of milk (agalactia) is better treated using drugs that stimulate mammary development such as domperidone.

• Oxytocin is frequently diluted in a liter of intravenous (IV) fluid for continuous slow infusion.

• Oxytocin is FDA approved in the horse, and it is a prescription drug. U.S. federal law restricts this drug to use by or on the lawful written or oral order of a licensed veterinarian within the context of a valid veterinarian-client-patient relationship.

Special Populations

Breeding Animals

Oxytocin is a hormone specifically used to treat uterine and lacta-tion problems in the mare. Oxytocin would not be commonly used in stallions.

Foals

Oxytocin is not used in foals.

Ponies

Pony breeds do not appear to differ from horses in their response to oxytocin.

Geriatrics

Oxytocin is not used in older animals, except in the context of breeding management.

Competition Horses

Oxytocin is not commonly used in competition horses. It would be forbidden in any drug-free competition, but it may not be regulated under many types of rules. It is important to check with the individual regulatory group.

Dose and Route of Administration

Injectable:

> 0.5 IU to 20 IU/1,000 lb, given IM or IV. May be repeated every 20 to 30 minutes.

> 80 to 100 IU diluted in 1 liter of intravenous fluid, administered slowly, IV

There is a wide range of doses and a variety of protocols for oxytocin use.

Dose Form: Injectable: 10 USP units/ml and 20 USP units/ml

AT A GLANCE:

PENICILLIN ANTIBIOTICS

GENERIC NAME	COMMON BRAND NAME
Ampicillin	Amp-Equine
Benzathine penicillin G	Ambi-Pen, Combicillin, Durapen, others
Procaine penicillin G	Crysticillin, Pfi-Pen G, Pen-G, others
Potassium penicillin G	Penicillin G potassium
Sodium penicillin B	Penicillin G sodium
Ticarcillin	Ticillin, Ticar

DRUG TYPE	INDICATIONS
Antibiotic	Susceptible bacterial infections

Basic Information

The discovery of penicillin in 1928 gave the world its first antibiotic and changed the course of medicine. Since then many different varieties of penicillin antibiotics have been created. The penicillins are bactericidal, which means they kill bacteria. They do this by destroying the bacteria's cell wall, and they are most effective against actively reproducing bacteria. The penicillins are some of the most commonly used antibiotics in veterinary medicine.

The different groups of penicillins can be distinguished by their effectiveness against different types of bacteria. The natural penicillins, which include the penicillin G antibiotics, work against *Streptococcus* and other Gram-positive bacteria. The aminopenicillins, such as ampicillin, are effective against a broader spectrum of bacteria, including some Gram-positives and Gram-negatives. Extended-spectrum penicillins include ticarcillin. These are active against a broad spectrum of bacteria, including *Pseudomonas*, which are often resistant to other antibiotics.

Some types of bacteria, including many species of *Staphylococcus*, produce an enzyme called penicillinase that inactivates penicillin.

Ticarcillin or amoxicillin combined with potassium clavulanate is frequently used to treat these difficult-to-control infections. These combinations are called potentiated penicillins.

Penicillins are widely distributed throughout most organs and tissues of the body shortly after administration. However, penetration into the central nervous system and eye occurs only when there is inflammation. This limits the drugs' usefulness for infections of these organs. Excretion occurs primarily through the kidneys and urine. When used in horses, penicillin antibiotics are injected intramuscularly (IM) or intravenously (IV). They are poorly absorbed when administered orally.

Side Effects, Precautions, and Overdose

• Hypersensitivity and serious side effects to penicillin are rare in animals. Penicillins should not be used in animals that have had an allergic reaction to any antibiotic in this group or to cephalosporin antibiotics because of the possibility of cross-reactivity.

• Procaine penicillin should not be given in the vein due to the procaine. Any leaks into blood vessels may be dangerous and can cause neurologic signs, convulsions, collapse, and even death. Although procaine reactions can occur even with careful injection technique, close attention to drawing back on the syringe while looking for blood will minimize this risk. Procaine reactions can be difficult to distinguish from allergic reactions.

• IV penicillin injections with potassium or sodium penicillin should be given very slowly to avoid collapse or neurologic side effects.

• Penicillin should not be given orally in horses. It is poorly absorbed and may cause diarrhea and colicky symptoms.

• IM penicillin injections can cause injection site reactions. These reactions usually respond to hot compresses and nonsteroidal anti-inflammatories (NSAIDs). Contact your veterinarian if you notice a reaction. Large volume injections increase the likelihood of an injection site reaction. Only 10 to 15 ml should be injected in each site.

• Very high doses or overdoses of penicillin may cause neurologic signs. Horses with decreased kidney function may be more likely to experience adverse effects.

Drug Interactions

• Penicillin antibiotics should not be combined with bacteriostatic antibiotics such as erythromycin, tetracycline, or neomycin.

• Ampicillin may affect the activity of rifampin.

• Large doses of certain penicillins, including ticarcillin, have been associated with bleeding problems in humans. They should be used cautiously in patients receiving oral anticoagulants or heparin.

Special Considerations

• IV penicillin, such as ampicillin or penicillin G potassium, is frequently used with aminoglycoside antibiotics to provide broad-spectrum coverage for severe mixed bacterial infections.

• Penicillin G sodium is very difficult to find and may only be available for emergency situations.

• Penicillin G potassium, ampicillin, and ticarcillin are used in the uterus of mares for the treatment of endometritis.

• Ampicillin comes in two forms: sodium and trihydrate. Sodium ampicillin is given IV or IM and is the generally recommended form of this drug.

• Benzathine penicillin is a combination product of benzathine and procaine penicillin. This product is designed as a long-acting penicillin that is given every two to three days rather than daily. It is not usually recommended in horses because blood levels do not remain high enough to be effective against many bacterial infections.

• Procaine penicillin and ampicillin are FDA approved in the horse and are prescription drugs. Ticarcillin is only labeled for intrauterine use but is commonly used systemically and its use is accepted practice. Neither Penicillin G sodium nor Penicillin G potassium is FDA approved in the horse, but each is commonly used and its use is accepted practice. U.S. federal law restricts these drugs to use by or on the lawful written or oral order of a licensed veterinarian within the context of a valid veterinarian-client-patient relationship.

Special Populations

Breeding Animals

Studies of laboratory animals have found that penicillins cross the placenta into the fetal blood. Birth defects and other adverse effects have not been reported, but these studies have not been repeated in the horse. Clinical experience in horses supports the work in other species. Penicillin is excreted in the milk of other species. This does not appear to cause clinical problems in nursing foals. Ticarcillin is frequently used in semen extenders for breeding stallions.

Foals

The penicillin antibiotics are among the safest antibiotics to use in foals. Penicillin is excreted by the kidneys. Foals with decreased kidney function should be monitored carefully, and lower doses may be indicated. Very young foals are able to partially absorb some oral penicillin. They lose that ability by one to three weeks of age.

Ponies

Pony breeds do not appear to differ from horses in their response to penicillin.

Geriatrics

The penicillin antibiotics are among the safest drugs to use in older animals. Penicillin is excreted by the kidneys. Horses with decreased kidney function should be monitored carefully, and lower doses may be indicated.

Competition Horses

Penicillin antibiotics are not permitted in drug-free competitions, but many regulatory groups do not prohibit antibiotics. Except procaine and benzathine penicillin, the penicillin antibiotics are not restricted for horses showing under USEF's therapeutic substance rules.

The use of procaine penicillin or benzathine penicillin is a common cause of drug violations in competition horses because procaine is chemically related to drugs that are used to mask pain. Procaine can be detected for 18 to 30 days, depending on the sensitivity of the test. Consult with the individual regulatory agency for more specific information.

Dose and Route of Administration

Injectable:

Ampicillin: 5 to 7 mg/lb, IV or IM, three to four times a day

Benzathine penicillin: 5,000 to 20,000 IU/lb, IM only, once every two to three days

Procaine penicillin: 10,000 to 22,000 IU/lb, IM only, two to three times a day

Penicillin G potassium: 5,000 to 22,000 IU/lb, IV or IM (usually given IV), four times a day

Penicillin G sodium: 5,000 to 22,000 IU/lb, IV or IM (usually given IV), four times a day

Ticarcillin: 20 to 40 mg/lb, IV or IM, three times a day

Dose Form:

Ampicillin: 1 and 3 gram vials to be reconstituted

Benzathine penicillin: 300,000 IU/ml in 100 ml and 250 ml bottles

Procaine penicillin: 300,000 IU/ml in 100 ml and 250 ml bottles

Penicillin G potassium: 5 million, 10 million, and 20 million IU vials to be reconstituted

Penicillin G sodium: 5 million IU vials to be reconstituted

Ticarcillin: 6, 20, and 30 gram vials to be reconstituted

Basic Information

Pergolide is a drug used in humans for the treatment of Parkinson's disease and the drug of choice for the treatment of pituitary pars intermedia dysfunction in horses. Pergolide works by binding with drug receptors in the brain that control the production of dopamine (a chemical called a neurotransmitter, produced by the brain).

For many years pituitary pars intermedia dysfunction was called pituitary adenoma. This is no longer thought to be technically correct. In most cases pituitary pars intermedia dysfunction is caused by enlargement or hypertrophy of the pituitary gland; only rarely is there actually a tumor. Because animals with pituitary pars intermedia dysfunction usually have clinical signs similar to Cushing's disease in humans, this condition may also be called equine Cushing's-like disease (ECD). Regardless of the name, this is a common problem of the older horse or pony.

Pituitary pars intermedia dysfunction is a medical problem that is managed, not cured. Animals that are being treated are usually on medication for the rest of their lives.

Side Effects, Precautions, and Overdose

• No information was found on side effects from pergolide therapy in the horse. A number of side effects are listed in humans taking pergolide along with other medication for Parkinson's disease. Side effects include low blood pressure, headache, gastrointestinal (GI) upset, anemia, respiratory infections, dizziness, and hallucinations.

• Overdose in humans causes GI upset and hallucinations.

Drug Interactions

• Phenothiazine tranquilizers such as acepromazine may interfere with the action of pergolide.

Special Considerations

• Pergolide is considered the drug of choice for pituitary pars intermedia dysfunction.

• Cyproheptadine is another drug that is used to treat this problem.

• Horses are usually started on a low dose (0.5 mg/day). Clinical response should be evaluated after one or two months. Improvement of clinical signs usually occurs by six weeks. If there is no improvement, the dose should be gradually increased (by 0.25 mg) until improvement is seen.

• It is important to identify and use the lowest possible dose of pergolide. There is some thought that this condition over time may become resistant to medication.

• Although pergolide is not FDA approved for use in horses, it is commonly used and considered accepted practice to do so. It is a prescription drug. U.S. federal law restricts this drug to use by or on the lawful written or oral order of a licensed veterinarian within the context of a valid veterinarian-client-patient relationship.

Special Populations

Breeding Animals

High doses of pergolide have been tested in laboratory animals without causing detectable harm to the fetus. This work has not been done in horses. It is not known if pergolide is excreted in milk, but this type of drug may interfere with lactation. Pergolide should only be used in pregnant or lactating animals if the benefits outweigh the risks. No information was found on pergolide use in breeding stallions.

Foals

No information was found on pergolide use in foals. It is hard to imagine the circumstances when it would be indicated.

Ponies

Pony breeds do not appear to differ from horses in their response to pergolide.

Geriatrics

Pergolide is commonly used in older horses and ponies.

Competition Horses

Pergolide is prohibited or regulated in most sanctioned competitions. Oral drugs are much more likely to have variable detection times. Long-term or repeated doses can also affect detection times. USEF has provisions in its rules for the therapeutic use of prohibited substances. Consult your veterinarian and the individual regulatory group if you are competing with a horse receiving pergolide.

Dose and Route of Administration

Oral: 0.5 to 2.0 mg per day

Dose Form: 0.25, 1.0 mg tablets, multiple formulations from compounding pharmacies

AT A GLANCE:

PHENYLBUTAZONE

GENERIC NAME
Phenylbutazone

COMMON BRAND NAME
Equiphen, Butatabs,
Phenylzone

DRUG TYPE
Nonsteroidal anti-inflammatory
drug

INDICATIONS
Pain relief particularly for
musculoskeletal pain,
anti-inflammatory, fever
reduction

Basic Information

Phenylbutazone is a nonsteroidal anti-inflammatory drug (NSAID). It is a potent pain reliever, fever reducer, and anti-inflammatory. Phenylbutazone is frequently prescribed for lameness, musculoskeletal pain from soft tissue injury, muscle soreness, bone and joint problems, and laminitis.

NSAIDs are used for musculoskeletal pain because they both relieve pain and decrease inflammation. They do not speed healing or cure the underlying problem, but they can make the horse more comfortable while he is recovering. Phenylbutazone and other NSAIDs are also frequently prescribed to reduce or control fevers due to viral or bacterial infections. These drugs only provide symptomatic relief by lowering the fever. They do not treat the underlying infection, and they can mask the severity of the problem if used without appropriate veterinary evaluation and therapy.

NSAIDs work by inhibiting the body's production of prostaglandins and other chemicals that stimulate the body's inflammatory response. Some of their actions may be dose dependent. NSAIDs are quickly absorbed into the blood stream; pain relief and fever reduction usually start within one to two hours.

Phenylbutazone is an inexpensive, generally well-tolerated drug. It is frequently the first choice for pain control of many musculoskeletal problems. Other NSAIDs, such as flunixin, are more commonly used for gastrointestinal (GI) pain or colic.

Recent research into NSAID toxicity and equine gastric ulcer disease may have given phenylbutazone a bad reputation for safety. When used at the appropriate dose and according to directions, phenylbutazone is generally a safe and an effective drug. Additional care should be shown with special populations such as foals, ponies, older horses, and debilitated or dehydrated horses. These populations are more likely to have adverse side effects.

Side Effects, Precautions, and Overdose

• The most common side effects include ulceration of the mouth and GI tract.

• Rare side effects include kidney damage, bleeding disorders, and protein loss.

• Injection site reactions can occur if blood leaks back at the injection site. Injectable phenylbutazone is very irritating to tissue if any leaks out of the vein. Do not inject in the muscle, under the skin, or intra-arterially.

• NSAIDs should be avoided or very carefully monitored in horses with liver disease, kidney disease, or GI problems.

• Overdoses of phenylbutazone can cause GI ulcers, protein loss, kidney and liver damage, and death. Early signs of toxicity include loss of appetite, ulcers in the mouth, and depression.

Drug Interactions

• Avoid combining with other anti-inflammatory drugs that tend to cause GI ulcers, such as corticosteroids and other NSAIDs.

• Avoid combining with anticoagulant drugs, particularly coumarin derivatives such as warfarin.

Special Considerations

• Some veterinarians may use more than one NSAID in combination, for example, flunixin and phenylbutazone given together. This is sometimes called stacking. Although there is little experimental evidence to support this practice, the theory is that different NSAIDs may act differently on different body systems. Particular care needs to be taken in this situation to avoid additive toxicity.

• Phenylbutazone is FDA approved in the horse, and it is a prescription drug. U.S. federal law restricts this drug to use by or on the lawful written or oral order of a licensed veterinarian within the context of a valid veterinarian-client-patient relationship.

Special Populations

Breeding Animals

Work in other species indicates that phenylbutazone may be harmful to the embryo. The drug can cross the placenta and is found in milk. These studies have not been repeated in the horse, but phenylbutazone should be used with caution in pregnant or nursing mares. No adverse effects on sperm production have been reported.

Foals

Phenylbutazone may be used in foals, but it should be used with particular caution to avoid GI ulceration and maintain kidney function. Premature foals, septicemic foals, foals with questionable kidney or liver function, and foals with diarrhea require careful monitoring. Drugs to protect the GI tract such as omeprazole, cimetidine, and sucralfate are frequently used with phenylbutazone.

Ponies

Pony breeds may be more susceptible to side effects from NSAIDs than horses. This is particularly true for phenylbutazone. When NSAIDs are used in ponies, the drug should be used with caution and at the lowest effective dose.

Geriatrics

Older horses, especially those with decreased kidney or liver function, may be more at risk for side effects. When phenylbutazone is used in older horses, it should be used carefully and at the lowest effective dose.

Competition Horses

Phenylbutazone is either a regulated or prohibited substance in most sanctioned competitions. It is a prohibited class A medication under the new FEI rules. USEF has a lengthy discussion of phenylbutazone and other NSAIDs in its drug rules. Phenylbutazone may be detected in blood or urine samples for up to seven days, depending on the sensitivity of the test. Many regulatory groups have a permissible drug detection level. Phenylbutazone is a common cause of positive drug tests both because it is a commonly used drug and because its metabolism can vary among horses, especially with oral use.

Dose and Route of Administration

Oral: 1 to 2 mg/lb, twice a day

Injectable: 1 to 2 mg/lb, twice a day, IV only

Dose Form:

Oral: 1 gram tablets, 6 or 12 gram paste syringe, 4 gram gel syringe

Injectable: 200 mg/ml

AT A GLANCE:

POLYSULFATED GLYCOSAMINOGLYCAN

GENERIC NAME
Polysulfated glycosaminoglycan,
PSGAG

COMMON BRAND NAME
Adequan

DRUG TYPE
Disease-modifying osteo-
arthritis agent, cartilage
protective agent

INDICATIONS
Non-infectious, degener-
ative, and/or traumatic
arthritis

Basic Information

Polysulfated glycosaminoglycan is a drug that is thought to protect cartilage, decrease inflammation in joints, and slow the progression of arthritis. It is chemically very similar to glycosaminoglycan, the principal component of cartilage and joint fluid. PSGAG is injected in the muscle or directly into a joint to treat some joint problems and lameness.

Normal joints have pads of cartilage protecting the ends of the bones that form the joint and a surrounding capsule lined by a synovial membrane. This membrane is very active in maintaining healthy joint function. Among its functions is the production of the lubricating joint fluid that helps reduce friction and wear on the joint surfaces. Glycosaminoglycans (GAGs), a group of organic chemicals composed of protein and carbohydrate molecules, make up a large percentage of the cartilage, joint fluid, and synovial membrane. The most common GAGs of joints are the unsulfonated GAG hyaluronic acid (HA) and several sulfonated GAGs, including chondroitin and glucosamine. GAGs are manufactured by the chondrocytes (cells that manufacture cartilage). The synovial lining of the joint also manufactures HA.

Joint injury starts a cycle of inflammation, cartilage damage, and poor quality joint fluid that ultimately leads to irreversible degeneration and degenerative joint disease. One of the earliest signs of joint damage or degenerative joint disease is the loss of GAGs from the cartilage within the joint. PSGAG is thought to protect cartilage by inhibiting enzymes that break down cartilage, inhibiting prostaglandin, and decreasing inflammation. PSGAG may also stimulate the cells that rebuild cartilage and produce joint fluid.

PSGAG is distributed throughout the body after intramuscular (IM) administration. It is found in all tissues and joints within two hours with the highest levels occurring in inflamed joints. It reaches maximal levels 48 hours after injection and lasts for 72 hours. PSGAG that is not incorporated into tissues is excreted unchanged by the kidneys.

Side Effects, Precautions, and Overdose

• Side effects from IM injection are rare even when high doses are given. The most common side effect is pain at the injection site.

• Occasionally, joint injections of PSGAG cause an acute inflammatory reaction in the joint. In these cases it is important to differentiate between a drug reaction and an infected joint. As a precaution against infection, many veterinarians add antibiotics to the PSGAG when injecting a joint.

• Do not use in infected joints.

• PSGAG is a very safe drug. Experimental overdose of five times the recommended dose for six weeks caused no adverse effect.

Drug Interactions

• PSGAG is related to heparin. It should be used with caution in animals that are also being treated with anticoagulants.

Special Considerations

• The single most helpful treatment for any injured joint is rest. However, the use of anti-arthritic agents that protect and promote repair of cartilage in joints may be very desirable, especially when combined with other means of controlling inflammation. PSGAG reduces prostaglandin concentrations in the joint. Some clinicians feel that this anti-inflammatory action is the most important function of PSGAG.

• PSGAG is commonly prescribed after joint surgery.

• Hyaluronic acid or its salt, sodium hyaluronate, is another glycosaminoglycan product. It is licensed for intravenous and intra-articular use in horses. (See Hyaluronic Acid.)

• Oral GAGs are nutritional supplements. Most of these products contain chondroitin sulphate, glucosamine, or both. These products are sometimes called neutraceuticals, a term that was coined in recent years to describe a food supplement that might have medicinal properties. Chondroitin sulphate, dermaton sulphate, heparan sulphate, keratan sulphate, and hyaluronan are GAGs that are naturally found in joint cartilage. Glucosamine is a small molecule that is used by the cells that make cartilage in the production of glycosaminoglycan. These neutraceuticals are made from a variety of sources including green-lipped mussels and cattle and shark cartilage. At present there is very little independent research on these products. While some veterinarians believe in their use, others do not. There is a great deal of research being done in this area at this time, and more information should become available. There has been some variability in content and quality-control issues among different brands of oral GAG supplements. Many of these products are marketed as combinations and may also include methylsulfonyl methane (MSM), vitamins, and minerals.

• PSGAG is FDA approved in the horse and is a prescription drugs. U.S. federal law restricts this drug to use by or on the lawful written or oral order of a licensed veterinarian within the context of a valid veterinarian-client-patient relationship.

Special Populations

Breeding Animals

Reproductive studies have not been done. Use with caution in pregnant and lactating mares and in breeding stallions.

Foals

There are no specific contraindications to using this product in young animals.

Ponies

Pony breeds do not appear to differ from horses in their response to PSGAG.

Geriatrics

PSGAG is considered safe in senior animals.

Competition Horses

PSGAG is commonly used in competition horses. It is forbidden during drug-free competitions, such as during an FEI-level competition. USEF has provisions in its rules for the therapeutic use of prohibited substances; PSGAG is permitted in horses showing under the therapeutic substance rules. It is important to check with the individual regulatory group.

Dose and Route of Administration

Injectable:

Intramuscular: 500 mg once every three to four days for four to seven injections

Intra-articular: 250 mg once a week for five weeks

Dose Form: 100 and 250 mg/ml injectable

AT A GLANCE:

PONAZURIL

GENERIC NAME
Ponazuril

COMMON BRAND NAME
Marquis

DRUG TYPE
Anticoccidial
Antiprotozoal

INDICATIONS
Equine protozoal
myeloencephalitis

Basic Information

Ponazuril was the first FDA-approved treatment for equine protozoal myeloencephalitis. It is "an anticoccidial compound with cidal activity against several types of protozoal parasites, including *Sarcocystis neurona* which causes EPM." The term "cidal" means that this drug kills the parasite. Ponazuril crosses the blood/brain barrier so it is able to reach effective levels in the central nervous system (CNS) and kill the migrating parasite within the spinal cord. In trials at six referral clinics, nearly 60% of the 102 participating horses either improved in their neurologic status or converted to a negative cerebral spinal fluid tap (CSF).

Side Effects, Precautions, and Overdose

• Studies by the manufacturer and the referral clinics showed a low incidence of relatively mild side effects, including loose manure, occasional loss of appetite, weight loss, mild colic, blisters of the mouth and nose, skin rash, and hives.

• No specific information is available at this time regarding overdose. The manufacturer conducted safety trials at six times the recommended dose. This small group of horses had similar side effects and no major systemic failures.

Drug Interactions

• No information is available at this time regarding drug interactions.

Special Considerations

• The manufacturer emphasizes that although ponazuril will "effectively clear the horse of *S. neurona*, it may have no effect on irreparable, pre-existing CNS damage caused by the protozoal parasite prior to treatment." This is an important consideration. After a successful course of treatment, the horse may no longer have EPM, but it may remain neurologic because of permanent damage to the CNS.

• Relapse seems to be a problem for some horses after treatment with ponazuril and/or sulfamethoxazole (SMZ)/pyrimethamine. Veterinarians disagree about how to best treat this population.

• Many veterinarians increase the length of time of treatment from the recommended 28 days to 56 days.

• Ponazuril is FDA approved in the horse, and it is a prescription drug. U.S. federal law restricts this drug to use by or on the lawful written or oral order of a licensed veterinarian within the context of a valid veterinarian-client-patient relationship.

Special Populations

Breeding Animals

The safety of ponazuril in pregnant and lactating mares and in breeding stallions has not been determined. There is one published paper looking at treatment with ponazuril in a small group of stallions. In this group there were no adverse effects on sperm production. There are also anecdotal reports on small trials on pregnant mares, but none of this work has been published. This drug should only be used in breeding animals when the benefits clearly outweigh the potential risks.

Foals

Foals do not commonly develop EPM. This drug should only be used in foals when the benefits clearly outweigh the potential risks.

Ponies

Pony breeds are similar to horses in their response to ponazuril.

Geriatrics

No information is available concerning the use of ponazuril in older horses.

Competition Horses

Ponazuril would be prohibited in any drug-free competition, but some regulatory groups may not regulate this drug. It is important to check with the individual regulatory organization.

Dose and Route of Administration

Oral: 2.27 mg/lb, once a day for 28 days

Dose Form: Multidose paste syringes. Each syringe contains enough drug to treat a 1,200-lb horse for seven days.

AT A GLANCE:

PROGESTERONE

GENERIC NAME
Progesterone
Altrenogest

COMMON BRAND NAME
Progesterone in oil
Regu-Mate

DRUG TYPE
Hormone

INDICATIONS
Control of reproductive
cycle, pregnancy mainte-
nance, and behavior
modification

Basic Information

Progesterone is a sex hormone normally produced by a structure
on the ovary called the corpus luteum and by the placenta of pregnant mares. Altrenogest is a synthetic progestin, which has activity
similar to that of progesterone.

Progesterone and altrenogest are used for a variety of purposes in the
reproductive management of mares: to prevent mares from coming
into heat, to synchronize estrous cycles for better breeding efficiency, to
organize or regulate heat cycles during the mare's seasonal transition,
and to help maintain pregnancy. These drugs are also used to modify
estrous-related behaviors that interfere with performance and pleasure
riding in non-breeding mares and occasionally in stallions.

Side Effects, Precautions, and Overdose

• The most common side effects for progesterone in oil are injection site reactions such as pain and swelling. These reactions usually respond to hot compresses and NSAIDs. Contact your veterinarian if you notice a reaction.

• There are no recognized side effects reported in the horse for
altrenogest when used according to label directions.

• Progesterone in oil is for intramuscular (IM) injection only. Do
not inject intravenously (IV).

• PRECAUTIONS FOR HUMANS: Altrenogest has some very serious potential side effects that can occur in humans who handle or
administer this drug. Read the package insert for precautions and

handling instructions. The manufacturer of Regu-Mate lists a number of groups, including pregnant women; people with heart, vascular, or liver diseases; and people with certain types of cancer, who should not be exposed to this drug. Rubber gloves should be worn when handling this product.

- Progesterone compounds, including altrenogest, should not be used in mares with chronic uterine infections.

- The long-term use of progesterone compounds may delay the return to normal reproductive cycling in mares.

Drug Interactions

- Rifampin may increase the speed of metabolism of administered progesterone compounds. This interaction is unlikely to occur often because rifampin is primarily used to treat *Rhodococcus equi* infections of foals and progesterones are generally used for reproductive management of broodmares.

Special Considerations

- Many progesterone in oil compounds are formulated and marketed by private pharmacies.

- Progesterone is sometimes combined with estrogen, another ovarian hormone, and used for many of the same purposes. This product is frequently called "P+" or "P and E."

- Altrenogest is FDA approved for use in the horse. Progesterone in oil is not FDA approved, but it is commonly used and accepted practice. Progesterone in oil and altrenogest are prescription drugs. U.S. federal law restricts these drugs to use by or on the lawful written or oral order of a licensed veterinarian within the context of a valid veterinarian-client-patient relationship.

Special Populations

Breeding Animals

Injectable progesterone is commonly used and accepted as safe in the pregnant mare. Although the manufacturer's label specifically says not to use altrenogest in pregnant mares, it is one of the more common and accepted uses. Progesterone and altrenogest are frequently used in mares with foals at foot with no apparent effect on the foal. Altrenogest is used occasionally on unruly stallions in an effort to calm them. There is little research regarding the effects of progesterone compounds on stallions, but there may be some detrimental effects from altrenogest use in younger stallions. Consult with your veterinarian.

Foals

It would be unusual to use progesterone in the foal, and no research is available to determine the risk.

Ponies

Pony breeds are similar to horses in their response to progesterone compounds.

Geriatrics

Progesterone compounds would not be commonly used in geriatric horses.

Competition Horses

Progesterone compounds would be forbidden in any drug-free competition, but they may not be regulated under many types of rules. Altrenogest is now permitted in mares at FEI competitions. It is important to check with the individual regulatory body.

Dose and Route of Administration

Oral: Altrenogest: 0.01ml/lb

Injectable: There are many different regimens for injectable progesterone depending on the intended use: 150 mg to 300 mg, IM, once a day, is a common dose.

Dose Form:

Oral: Altrenogest, 0.22% solution

Injectable: Progesterone in oil, 100 mg/ml and 50 mg/ml

Basic Information

Prostaglandins are a group of substances produced in many locations throughout the body. Naturally occurring prostaglandins have many biological functions in addition to their role in reproduction. Synthetic prostaglandin is given to mares primarily to manipulate their heat or estrous cycle. It also is used to terminate pregnancy and to treat uterine infections.

The estrous cycle is divided into different phases. During estrus, the mare is in "heat" and receptive to the stallion. Toward the end of estrus, ovulation occurs and a mature egg is released from within a follicle. After ovulation, the follicle develops into a structure called the corpus luteum (CL), which produces progesterone. This phase of the estrous cycle is called diestrus; progesterone is the dominant hormone, and the mare is no longer receptive to the stallion. After about 14 days, if the mare is not pregnant, the mare's uterus will normally produce enough prostaglandin to "lyse" or terminate the CL and she will return to heat. Prostaglandin controls the lifespan of the CL, and by doing so, controls the length of the estrous cycle.

Prostaglandin may be given to shorten the diestrous phase of the estrous cycle. This is often referred to as short-cycling. Prostaglandin may also be used to restart cycling in a mare with a prolonged diestrous phase or to terminate an early pregnancy. For prostaglandin to work, the mare must have a mature CL that is actively producing progesterone. Generally, the CL reaches maturity four or five days after the mare goes out of heat. That is the reason veterinarians want the mare to tease "cold" or be unreceptive for five days before giving prostaglandin. There is some variation in how fast a mare will return to heat and ovulate after prostaglandin is given. Rectal palpation or ultrasound of the ovaries before administering prostaglandin may be helpful. If the mare has a big follicle already present on the ovary she may return to heat and ovulate faster than the mare with no palpable follicle.

Prostaglandin is also used in the treatment of uterine infections, endometritis, and pyometra, a severe uterine infection involving the accumulation of inflammatory fluid in the uterus. Uterine infections are easier to diagnose and treat during estrus. In addition, the mare's immune system can fight infection better when the mare is in heat.

Side Effects, Precautions, and Overdose

• Because prostaglandins affect many body systems, side effects are common. They may be quite dramatic but usually are not life-threatening. Side effects usually diminish in 30 to 60 minutes. Common side effects may be restlessness, cramping, sweating, colic-like pain, panting, high heart rate, diarrhea, urination, and defecation.

• PRECAUTIONS FOR HUMANS: Pregnant women, asthmatics, or persons with bronchial disease should not handle this product. Any accidental exposure to skin should be washed off immediately.

• Prostaglandin is for intramuscular (IM) injection only. Do not inject intravenously (IV).

• Signs of overdose are the same as the side effects, but more severe.

Drug Interactions

• Prostaglandins may enhance the activity of other drugs that affect the uterus, such as oxytocin.

Special Considerations

• For prostaglandin to be effective in bringing a mare into heat, she must have a functional CL that is producing progesterone. If a mare is not responding to prostaglandin treatment, it may be worthwhile to check her progesterone level as a part of an overall reproductive work up.

• The term "shut-down" is sometimes used to describe mares with small, firm, inactive ovaries. These mares usually do not have circulating progesterone and may not respond to prostaglandin. Mares can "shut down" due to a variety of reasons, including season, hormone treatments, ovarian tumors, and age.

• Mares are seasonal breeders. In the winter they stop cycling and go into "seasonal anestrus." Mares in anestrus will not respond to prostaglandin because they do not have a CL. As spring comes and day length increases, these mares will naturally begin to cycle again.

• Mares that have been given high levels of anabolic steroids and other hormones may not respond to prostaglandin until their bodies are no longer under the effects of these drugs and they resume cycling.

• Prostaglandin will lyse the CL about 80% of the time.

• Many programs for estrous synchronization or regulation use prostaglandin at the end of a 10- or 12-day course of progesterone or altrenogest.

• A single dose of prostaglandin will effectively terminate an early pregnancy. It is much harder to terminate the pregnancy once the placenta forms "endometrial cups" and starts to produce progesterone. This occurs about 35 days after ovulation. Multiple doses of prostaglandin may be necessary or another method of termination may be required.

• Prostaglandin F2 alpha is FDA approved for use in the horse, and it is a prescription drug. U.S. federal law restricts this drug to use by or on the lawful written or oral order of a licensed veterinarian within the context of a valid veterinarian-client-patient relationship.

Special Populations

Breeding Animals

Prostaglandins should not be given to pregnant animals unless abortion is the desired result. Prostaglandin is frequently given to lactating mares with foals at foot with no apparent effects on the foal. Prostaglandin would not be commonly used in stallions.

Foals

Prostaglandin would not be commonly used in foals.

Ponies

Pony breeds are similar to horses in their response to prostaglandin.

Geriatrics

Prostaglandin would not be commonly used in older horses except older broodmares.

Competition Horses

Prostaglandin would not be commonly used in competition horses. It would be forbidden in any drug-free competition, but it may not be regulated under many types of competition rules. It is important to check with the individual regulatory group.

Dose and Route of Administration

Injectable: Prostaglandin F2 alpha: 5 to 10 mg, IM, or 1 mg/100 lbs body weight, IM

Dose Form: 5 mg/ml injectable

AT A GLANCE:

PYRIMETHAMINE

GENERIC NAME
Pyrimethamine
Pyrimethamine/Sulfadiazine

COMMON BRAND NAME
Daraprim
Rebalance

DRUG TYPE
Folic acid antagonist

INDICATIONS
Equine protozoal
myeloencephalitis

Basic Information

Pyrimethamine is an antiprotozoal drug that is used in combination with a sulfa antibiotic, generally sulfadiazine or sulfamethoxazole, for the treatment of equine protozoal myeloencephalitis (EPM). Pyrimethamine blocks a step in the metabolism of the protozoa by inhibiting an enzyme in the synthesis of folic acid, while the sulfa drug blocks a different step in the protozoa's folic acid synthesis. These drugs combined have a synergistic effect against *Sarcocystis neurona*, the protozoa that cause EPM. This drug combination does not kill the protozoa; it only inhibits further growth or reproduction. Pyrimethamine alone is not considered effective for the treatment of EPM. There is now an FDA-approved combination product of sulfadiazine and pyrimethamine available. Prior to the availability of the combination product, veterinarians prescribed pyrimethamine combined with the antibiotic trimethoprim-sulfa or SMZ-TMP.

Side Effects, Precautions, and Overdose

• Pyrimethamine should be used with extreme caution in animals with blood or bone marrow problems. The combination of pyrimethamine and sulfa may cause anemia, decreased platelets, decreased white blood cell counts, and suppressed bone marrow.

• Other uncommon side effects may include loss of appetite, diarrhea, and depression or lethargy.

• A treatment crisis or temporary worsening of neurologic symptoms can occur in animals treated with pyrimethamine/sulfa. This is thought to be due to inflammation caused by dying parasites in the central nervous system.

• There was no information found on overdose of pyrimethamine in the horse.

Drug Interactions

• No drug interactions are listed for horses. Interestingly, the use of SMZ-TMP with pyrimethamine is not recommended in humans because of the risk of bone marrow suppression. This does not seem to be a common side effect in horses.

Special Considerations

• The diagnosis and treatment of EPM is a controversial and rapidly evolving field. A great deal of research effort is being focused on this disease. There are new drugs for the treatment of EPM including ponazuril and nitazoxanide. Both of these drugs work by killing the protozoa. Case selection, personal experience, and economics may help determine which drug is chosen for an individual horse.

• There are conflicting opinions among veterinarians regarding folic acid supplementation for horses on the combination of pyrimethamine/sulfa. The concern is that long-term use of these drugs might inhibit folic acid metabolism in the horse. Whether this is true has not been confirmed. Consult your veterinarian.

• Treatment for EPM with pyrimethamine/sulfa usually requires long-term treatment (12 to 24 weeks).

• Pyrimethamine is not FDA approved in the horse, but it is commonly used and accepted practice. The combination product is FDA approved. They are prescription drugs, and U.S. federal law restricts the use of these drugs by or on the lawful written or oral order of a licensed veterinarian.

Special Populations
Breeding Animals
Pyrimethamine has been shown to cause birth defects in other

species. Some veterinarians have reported cases where they thought this EPM treatment caused abortions or reproductive losses in mares. Pyrimethamine is excreted in the milk of other species. It should only be used in pregnant or lactating mares when the benefits outweigh the potential risks. Limited research on pyrimethamine/sulfa combination showed no adverse effect on semen in stallions.

Foals

It is unlikely that pyrimethamine would be indicated in young foals because EPM is not likely to occur in foals.

Ponies

Pony breeds do not appear to differ from horses in their response to pyrimethamine.

Geriatrics

Pyrimethamine should be safe to use in older horses. The package insert cautions against using this drug in humans with decreased kidney or liver function.

Competition Horses

It is unlikely that competition horses would be receiving treatment for EPM while actively competing. Pyrimethamine would be prohibited in any drug-free competition, but some regulatory groups may not regulate this drug or have established a permissible blood level. It is important to check with the individual regulatory organization.

Dose and Route of Administration

Oral: 0.5 mg/lb, once a day

Dose Form: 25 mg tablets

AT A GLANCE:

RESERPINE

GENERIC NAME
Reserpine

COMMON BRAND NAME
Generics

DRUG TYPE
Long-acting tranquilizer/
sedative

INDICATIONS
Sedation

Basic Information

Reserpine is used as a long-acting tranquilizer in horses. It is used to sedate excitable or difficult horses that are laid up or on enforced rest, and it is sometimes used illicitly for the sedation of show horses and sale horses or in other circumstances where a "quieter" horse might be desired. Until relatively recently, reserpine was difficult to test for, but there are now accurate tests.

Reserpine was first isolated in 1952 from *Rauwolfia serpentina* or *Rauwolfia vomitoria*, plants found in India and Africa. In traditional herbal medicine, it is brewed as a tea. It was used primarily in humans to treat high blood pressure, insanity, snakebite, and cholera.

Reserpine works by blocking the storage of some of the brain's chemical messengers, especially a neurotransmitter called norepinephrine. It is a very unusual drug in that it takes many hours to days to reach full effect and continues to have some subtle sedating effects for many days after the last dose.

Side Effects, Precautions, and Overdose

• Reserpine can have some marked and dramatic side effects. Different horses vary greatly in their sensitivity to this drug.

• Common side effects include colic, gastrointestinal upset, mild diarrhea that may last for days, and sweating over the back and hind legs. Signs of sedation include depression, droopy eyes, and a dropped penis.

• Reserpine increases gastric secretion in humans and increases the risk of ulcers.

• Overdose of reserpine increases the risk and the severity of the aforementioned side effects.

Drug Interactions

• Reserpine may interact with drugs used for general anesthesia. It is important to keep accurate records of reserpine and any other medications used if an animal is referred to an equine hospital for intensive care or surgery.

• The antidote to reserpine is methamphetamine.

Special Considerations

• There is very little information published on the clinical use of reserpine in horses. Much of the available information is anecdotal and should be considered as such.

• Reserpine is not FDA approved in the horse. It is a prescription drug. U.S. federal law restricts this drug to use by or on the lawful written or oral order of a licensed veterinarian within the context of a valid veterinarian-client-patient relationship.

Special Populations

Breeding Animals

No information was found. Because reserpine causes male horses to drop their penises, penile paralysis in stallions is a possible side effect.

Foals

No information was found.

Ponies

No information was found.

Geriatrics

No information was found.

Competition Horses

Reserpine is a prohibited substance in most sanctioned competitions and is a frequent cause of drug violations. Most regulatory groups do not have a permitted threshold level. The amount and route of the dose, number of doses, and sensitivity of the test may affect detection. An article on the USEF Web site about drug rules suggests 90 days between the last dose of reserpine and any USEF competition. Some herbal products have been implicated in positive tests for reserpine.

Dose and Route of Administration

Reserpine is given both orally and intravenously. Consult your veterinarian for dosing information.

Some generic formulations are available, and these formulations can be purchased from compounding pharmacies.

AT A GLANCE:

RIFAMPIN

GENERIC NAME
Rifampin

COMMON BRAND NAME
Rifadin, Rimactane

DRUG TYPE
Antibiotic

INDICATIONS
Susceptible bacterial
infections

Basic Information

Rifampin is an antibiotic used almost exclusively in combination with erythromycin for the treatment of *Rhodococcus equi* infections in foals. This drug is somewhat unusual as it is always used with another antibiotic. If rifampin is used without another antibiotic, the bacteria are rapidly able to develop resistance.

R. equi infection can cause both a respiratory and a gastrointestinal (GI) form of disease. The respiratory form is more common. Both forms can be difficult to diagnose and to treat. These bacteria tend to cause abscesses, and most antibiotics do not penetrate abscesses in a high enough concentration to be effective. Fatalities can occur even with prompt diagnosis and treatment. Rifampin is particularly valuable for the treatment of this difficult bacterial infection because of its excellent penetration of most tissues, including bone, cerebral spinal fluid, and abscesses.

Rifampin can be either bactericidal (kills the bacteria) or bacteriostatic (prevents the bacteria from reproducing), depending on the specific organism and the concentration of the drug.

Side Effects, Precautions, and Overdose

• Side effects are rare in the horse. In other species, signs of GI pain, rashes, and increased liver enzymes have been reported, especially with long-term use.

- Occasionally, foals on the combination of rifampin and erythromycin may develop diarrhea. All antibiotic-related diarrheas require prompt attention. Consult with your veterinarian immediately about treatment.
- Rifampin can cause orange or red discoloration of urine or other bodily fluids. This is not harmful.
- Rifampin should be used with caution in animals with decreased liver function.
- Overdose increases the risk and severity of the aforementioned side effects.

Drug Interactions

- Rifampin may increase the metabolism of some drugs that are also metabolized by the liver, including chloramphenicol, corticosteroids, and anticoagulants. None of these drugs is likely to be used with rifampin in the treatment of *R. equi*.

Special Considerations

- Depending on the antibiotic susceptibility pattern of the infection, rifampin is occasionally used with other antibiotics such as trimethoprim sulfa.
- Rifampin is not FDA approved in the horse, but it is commonly used and an accepted practice. It is a prescription drug. U.S. federal law restricts this drug to use by or on the lawful written or oral order of a licensed veterinarian within the context of a valid veterinarian-client-patient relationship.

Special Populations

Breeding Animals

It is unlikely that this drug would be used in pregnant mares or breeding stallions because it is generally used in the treatment of *R. equi* in foals. It has been used in pregnant women without reported problems.

Foals

This drug is commonly used along with erythromycin or other antibiotics for the treatment of *R. equi* in foals

Ponies

Pony breeds do not appear to differ from horses in their response to rifampin.

Geriatrics

It is unlikely that this drug would be used in older horses as it is generally used in the treatment of *R. equi* in foals.

Competition Horses

It is unlikely that this drug would be used in competition horses as it is generally used in the treatment of *R. equi* in foals. It would not be permitted in drug-free competitions, but many regulatory groups do not prohibit antibiotics. Rifampin is not restricted by USEF for horses showing under the therapeutic substance rules. It is important to check with the individual regulatory agency.

Dose and Route of Administration

Oral: 1 to 2 mg/lb, two times a day with erythromycin

Dose Form: 150 mg and 300 mg capsules

AT A GLANCE:

ROMIFIDINE

GENERIC NAME
Romifidine hydrochloride

COMMON BRAND NAME
Sedivet

DRUG TYPE
Sedative

INDICATIONS
Tranquilization and
pre-anesthetic

Basic Information

Romifidine is a newer tranquilizer or sedative that has been available for many years in Europe but only recently marketed in the United States. It is from the same chemical family as xylazine and detomidine (alpha-2-adrenoreceptor agonists). The degree of sedation with romifidine is generally thought to be somewhere between that of xylazine and detomidine. Romifidine provides a longer duration of action than either xylazine or detomidine when given at an equivalent dose and the horses appear less ataxic, or wobbly. For this reason some veterinarians like using romifidine during radiographs or lameness examinations. Although technically this family of drugs has some analgesic properties, romifidine is not thought to provide particularly good pain relief.

Romifidine is frequently combined with butorphanol for improved pain management. It is sometimes used as a pre-anesthetic drug either before injectable anesthesia or before gas inhalation anesthesia. Romifidine is given by injection in the vein (IV). It is not well absorbed orally.

Side Effects, Precautions, and Overdose

• Romifidine initially slows the heart rate and can change the heart rhythm in some horses (dropped beats).

• Romifidine causes a decrease in gastrointestinal motility. There have been reports of mild colic subsequent to the use of romifidine.

• Horses will drop their heads (not as much as with xylazine or detomidine) and appear very sedate. Some loss of coordination and sweating are common. With any form of sedation, horses can react suddenly and unexpectedly. Always work carefully around a sedated horse no matter how "asleep" it appears. Horses can and will respond to painful stimulation.

• Romifidine should not be used in horses with abnormal heart rhythms or heart disease. It should be used with "extreme caution" in horses with other major health problems including shock, severe respiratory disease, and severe liver and kidney problems.

• Romifidine reduces the body's ability to regulate its temperature.

• On rare occasions, an individual horse may have a paradoxical response (excitement rather than sedation) when given romifidine. This may also occur with other alpha-2-agonist drugs.

• Romifidine has been tested by the manufacturer at up to five times the recommended dose. Overdose causes heart arrhythmias, low blood pressure, and respiratory and central nervous system depression.

• Yohimbine can be used to reverse some of the effects of romifidine.

Drug Interactions

• Romifidine has additive effects when combined with other tranquilizers and general anesthetic drugs. Although these combinations are frequently used in veterinary practice, this should only be done by veterinarians who are experienced with the use of these drugs.

• Intravenous trimethoprim sulfa should not be used in horses sedated with romifidine.

• Chloramphenicol can interfere with the metabolism of alpha-2-agonist drugs.

Special Considerations

• Romifidine causes a drop in blood pressure, but to a lesser degree than acepromazine.

• When sedating a horse using romifidine, it is important to wait until the drug has taken effect before beginning any procedure. Sedation occurs two to four minutes after IV injection.

• Romifidine is FDA approved in the horse, and it is a prescription drug. U.S. federal law restricts this drug to use by or on the order of a licensed veterinarian within the context of a valid veterinarian-client-patient relationship.

Special Populations
Breeding Animals

The manufacturer has not studied romifidine in pregnant mares or stallions. Other alpha-2-agonists have been used extensively in pregnant mares without reported problems. There is research that shows that this group of drugs causes increased intrauterine pressure and increased uterine motility, but there was no increase in number of abortions. It is not known if romifidine is present in milk. Although stallions may relax and drop their penis when treated with romifidine, there are no reports of penile paralysis such as those with acepromazine.

Foals

Because alpha-2-agonists can lower the heart rate, cause changes in blood pressure, and slow breathing, romifidine should be used with caution and at the lowest effective dose in sick foals and very young foals. Additionally, these drugs can affect an animal's ability to regulate its temperature. When used in very young foals, the foal should remain in a temperature-controlled area until it has fully recovered.

Ponies

Pony breeds do not appear to differ from horses in their response to romifidine.

Geriatrics

Romifidine should be used with caution in older animals. Many veterinarians start at the lower end of the dose range. Reversal with yohimbine might also be considered to minimize side effects.

Draft Horses

Draft horse breeds may be particularly sensitive to most sedatives. Many veterinarians start at the lower end of the dose range.

Competition Horses

Romifidine is a prohibited substance in most sanctioned competitions. It is a prohibited class A medication under the new FEI rules. It may be detected for up to 72 hours. Detection may be affected by number of doses and the sensitivity of the test. The USEF has provisions in its rules for the therapeutic use of prohibited substances. It is important to check with the individual regulatory group.

Dose and Route of Administration

Injectable: 18-55 micrograms (ug)/lb or 40-120 ug/kg, IV

Dose Form: 10 mg/ml, injectable

AT A GLANCE:

SUCRALFATE

GENERIC NAME
Sucralfate

DRUG TYPE
Anti-ulcer

COMMON BRAND NAME
Carafate

INDICATIONS
Ulcers of the gastrointestinal tract

Basic Information

Sucralfate is used to treat or protect against some types of gastric ulcers by forming a protective "Band-Aid" coating over the injured mucosa (lining) of the stomach or small intestine. It is minimally absorbed systemically and therefore its effects are local rather than systemic. It does not affect gastric acid production.

Sucralfate is most effective on ulcers affecting the glandular part of the stomach rather than the non-glandular or squamous areas. This is important because ulcers in foals and adult horses often involve the squamous type of mucosa and require the use of other drugs in addition to or instead of sucralfate.

Other commonly used drugs for the management and prevention of equine gastric ulcers are omeprazole and the H_2 antagonists, cimetidine and ranitidine.

Side Effects, Precautions, and Overdose

• Sucralfate is the safest drug available to treat glandular mucosal ulcers. Constipation is occasionally reported in humans and dogs, and could occur in horses and foals.

• Because sucralfate is very poorly absorbed, difficulties due to overdose are unlikely.

Drug Interactions

• Sucralfate can decrease the absorption of many drugs. It should not be given within two hours of most other oral medication. Administration at the same time as the H_2 antagonists does not seem to interfere with either drug's activity and is acceptable.

Special Considerations

• Sucralfate is sometimes prescribed as a precaution with non-steroidal anti-inflammatory drugs (NSAIDs), corticosteroids, and other drugs that can cause stomach ulcers.

• After a diagnosis of ulcers, drugs such as sucralfate are usually prescribed for two to three weeks in order to give the ulcers time to heal.

• Sucralfate is not FDA approved in the horse, but it is commonly used and accepted practice. It is a prescription drug. U.S. federal law restricts this drug to use by or on the lawful written or oral order of a licensed veterinarian within the context of a valid veterinarian-client-patient relationship.

Special Populations

Breeding Animals

Sucralfate has not been tested in the horse. In laboratory animals high doses of sucralfate did not cause harm to the fetus. It is not known if sucralfate is excreted in the milk of mares. Significant levels in milk are very unlikely because the drug is very poorly absorbed.

Foals

Sucralfate is commonly used in foals.

Ponies

Ponies do not appear to differ from horses in their response to sucralfate.

Geriatrics

Sucralfate is safe in older horses.

Competition Horses

Sucralfate is prohibited in any drug-free competition. Individual regulatory groups may have permissible detection levels. Sucralfate is permitted by USEF for horses showing under the therapeutic substance rules. It is important to check with the individual regulatory group.

Dose and Route of Administration

Oral: 0.5 to 1.0 mg/lb, two to four times a day. Or 2 to 4 grams/1,000 lbs, two to four times a day

Dose Form: 1 gram tablets or 100 mg/ml liquid suspension

AT A GLANCE:

TETRACYCLINE ANTIBIOTICS

GENERIC NAME
Doxycycline
Oxytetracycline

COMMON BRAND NAME
Vibramycin
Liquamycin, LA200,
Terramycin

DRUG TYPE
Antibiotic

INDICATIONS
Infections caused by
susceptible bacteria or
microorganisms

Basic Information

Tetracycline antibiotics are a group of antibiotics that are effective against a wide variety of bacterial infections. These drugs are bacteriostatic. They interfere with the normal growth cycle of the invading bacteria and prevent them from reproducing. This allows the body's immune system to fight off the infection. Oxytetracycline is the most commonly used injectable tetracycline in the horse. Doxycycline is less commonly used, but it is available as an oral medication.

Oxytetracycline is the drug of choice for the treatment of Potomac Horse Fever (equine monocytic ehrlichiosis) and other diseases caused by *Ehrlichia* organisms. It is also used in combination with sulfa antibiotics to treat bacterial respiratory infections such as pneumonia or pleuritis, particularly in racehorses and foals.

Tetracyline is also available in topical preparations, including ointments for use in the eyes and on the skin.

Side Effects, Precautions, and Overdose

• Tetracycline antibiotics can cause gastrointestinal (GI) problems, especially diarrhea. Because antibiotic-related diarrheas can be very difficult to manage or even be fatal, some veterinarians are very hesitant to use these drugs.

• Oxytetracycline is very irritating to tissue if any of the drug leaks out of the vein during or after intravenous injection. Do not inject oxytetracycline in the muscle or under the skin.

• Oxytetracycline should be diluted and injected very slowly. Rapid intravenous injection can cause the horse to collapse. Some horses can have an allergic or anaphylactic type of reaction to oxytetracycline injection.

• Tetracycline antibiotics should be used with care in animals with liver disease or kidney disease. A tetracycline drug should not be used in dehydrated horses until they are re-hydrated.

• Tetracycline administration should be stopped in any horse that develops diarrhea. The horse should be isolated until the feces are cultured for *Salmonella*, a contagious and potentially life-threatening Gram-negative bacteria. Occasionally, a horse that is an asymptomatic carrier of *Salmonella* develops full-blown clinical disease following antibiotic administration. Any antibiotic can kill the normal bacteria in the GI tract. The decrease in normal bacteria allows pathogenic bacteria that are present in small numbers to proliferate and cause disease. Antibiotic-induced diarrhea should be treated aggressively.

Drug Interactions

• Tetracycline antibiotics can interfere with the action of bactericidal (bacteria-killing) antibiotics such as penicillin. Do not give your animal more than one antibiotic without specific instructions from your veterinarian.

• Antacids, sodium bicarbonate powder, mineral supplements, and multivitamins containing bismuth, calcium, zinc, magnesium, and iron can reduce the effectiveness of oral tetracycline antibiotics such as doxycycline by interfering with their absorption into the blood stream. Doses of antacid, mineral, and vitamin supplements or sodium bicarbonate should be separated from the antibiotic by at least two hours.

• Cimetidine, ranitidine, and other H_2 blockers may reduce the amount of oral tetracyclines absorbed in the blood stream, decreasing the effectiveness.

• Tetracycline antibiotics may increase the effect of anticoagulant drugs such as warfarin.

Special Considerations

• Injectable oxytetracycline is occasionally given in high doses to young foals born with contracted tendons. It is used in this instance because it rapidly binds calcium, allowing for muscle and tendon relaxation. Depending on the degree of contracture and the response, this treatment may need to be repeated every other day. Additional therapy such as splints, exercise changes, and physical therapy may also be helpful. Many veterinarians think that this treatment is most effective in the very young foal with congenitally contracted tendons. It may be less effective in older foals. This treatment is not used in adult horses. It is important that the foal's kidneys are functioning well and that kidney function is monitored before and during high dose tetracycline therapy.

• Potomac Horse Fever (PHF) is one of the few instances when oxytetracycline is used in a horse that presents with diarrhea. Tetracyclines usually are considered a poor choice for horses with diarrhea because of the possible risk of *Salmonella*. The decision to begin treatment with oxytetracycline can be difficult because one may need to start antibiotic therapy before arriving at a positive diagnosis (bloodwork for PHF and fecal cultures for *Salmonella*). If the horse responds to the oxytetracycline, a diagnosis of PHF or another *Ehrlichia* organism may be made even before the bloodwork comes back.

• Oxytetracycline and doxycycline are not FDA approved in the horse, but they are commonly used and an accepted practice. They are prescription drugs. U.S. federal law restricts these drugs to use by or on the lawful written or oral order of a licensed veterinarian within the context of a valid veterinarian-client-patient relationship.

Special Populations

Breeding Animals

Tetracycline antibiotics cross the placenta and are present in milk. They can retard bone growth in the fetus and discolor teeth. They should be avoided unless the benefits outweigh the risks.

Foals

Tetracycline antibiotics are used for respiratory disease in older foals. Intravenous tetracycline is used in young foals for contracted tendons. (See Special Considerations.) Because intravenous tetracycline is irritating if any leaks out of the vein, and because of the necessity of slow injection and the difficulties involved in restraining foals, many veterinarians use an IV catheter when treating foals with this drug.

Ponies

Pony breeds do not appear to differ from horses in their response to tetracycline antibiotics.

Geriatrics

Tetracycline antibiotics can be used with care in older patients with normal kidney and liver function.

Competition Horses

Tetracycline antibiotics are not permitted in drug-free competitions, but many regulatory groups do not prohibit antibiotics or have established a permissible blood level. They are not restricted by USEF for horses showing under the therapeutic substance rules. It is important to check with the individual regulatory agency.

Dose and Route of Administration

Oral: Doxycycline:1.5 to 4.5 mg/lb, twice a day

Injectable: Oxytetracycline: 2 to 10 mg/lb, IV only, once or twice a day

Dose Form:

Doxycycline: 50 and 100 mg capsules and tablets

Oxytetracycline: 100 mg/ml and 200 mg/ml

AT A GLANCE:

TRICHLORMETHIAZIDE AND DEXAMETHASONE BOLUS

GENERIC NAME
Trichlormethiazide and
dexamethasone bolus

COMMON BRAND NAME
Naquasone/Compounded

DRUG TYPE
Diuretic and corticosteroid
combination

INDICATIONS
Non-specific swelling
or edema

Basic Information

Trichlor/dex is an oral combination product that was licensed and marketed under the name of Naquasone as a treatment for udder edema in the cow. It is no longer manufactured by the original company and may only be purchased through a compounding pharmacy. It is used in horses to reduce mild swellings, particularly of the legs. Trichlor/dex contains the diuretic trichlormethiazide and the corticosteroid dexamethasone. Trichlormethiazide causes the body to lose water and sodium chloride by decreasing the re-absorption of these electrolytes in the kidney. It has little effect on potassium excretion. Dexamethasone is a potent anti-inflammatory. The anti-inflammatory effects and side effects associated with dexamethasone are discussed in the monograph on corticosteroids. Because this is a combination product, and each component works by a different mechanism, trichlor/dex contains a smaller dose of the individual drugs than might be used if either drug were given alone.

Side Effects, Precautions, and Overdose

• Trichlor/dex can mask the signs of infection because of the corticosteroid's anti-inflammatory action.

• Trichlor/dex should not be used when a bacterial infection is present or suspected without treating the infection with appropriate antibiotic therapy.

• Dexamethasone is a corticosteroid. All of the potential side effects of corticosteroids should be reviewed and considered. Corticosteroids should not be used or used with extreme caution in any horse that is prone to laminitis.

• Trichlormethiazide, as a diuretic, causes the loss of water and sodium chloride. Electrolyte depletion and dehydration are possible with prolonged use or overdose. Free access to water and salt are important at all times.

Drug Interactions

• Trichlor/dex should not be used at the same time as other corticosteroids or diuretics.

Special Considerations

• Trichlor/dex does not cure the underlying cause of the swelling or edema and should not be used without appropriate diagnostic evaluation.

• Trichlor/dex is not FDA approved in the horse. It is commonly used and an accepted practice, and it is a prescription drug. U.S. federal law restricts this drug to use by or on the lawful written or oral order of a licensed veterinarian.

Special Populations

Breeding Animals

Corticosteroids are generally not recommended in pregnant animals. In some species corticosteroids may cause premature labor and birth defects. This has not been demonstrated in the horse. The drugs contained in trichlor/dex are excreted in milk. Trichlor/dex should not be used in pregnant or lactating mares unless the benefits outweigh the risks.

Foals

Trichlor/dex bolus would rarely be used in foals because steroids and diuretics are rarely used in foals, and it is difficult to divide the bolus to provide a small enough dose.

Ponies

Pony breeds may be more susceptible to some side effects from corticosteroids, particularly laminitis.

Geriatrics

Trichlor/dex is safe for use in older horses without major health problems. Trichlor/dex should not be used in horses with pituitary pars intermedia dysfunction (equine Cushing's-like syndrome, or pituitary hypertrophy/adenoma).

Competition Horses

Trichlor/dex is prohibited in any drug free competition, though individual regulatory groups may have permissible detection levels. It is a prohibited class A medication under the new FEI rules. It is important to check with the individual regulatory body. Dexamethasone may be detected in urine for approximately 24 to 48 hours depending on the sensitivity of the test.

Dose and Route of Administration

Oral: 200 mg trichlormethiazide combined with 5 mg dexamethasone given once a day in an adult horse. May be followed by a half-dose once a day.

Dose Form: Paste or powder containing 200 mg trichlormethiazide and 5 mg dexamethasone.

AT A GLANCE:

TRIMETHOPRIM SULFA

GENERIC NAME
Trimethoprim Sulfadiazine,
Trimethoprim Sulfamethoxazole,
SMZ-TMP

COMMON BRAND NAME
Di-Trim, Tribrissen

DRUG TYPE
Antibiotic

INDICATIONS
Susceptible bacterial
infections

Basic Information

Trimethoprim sulfa or SMZ-TMP is currently the most commonly used antibiotic in the horse. This type of antibiotic is called a potentiated sulfonamide. SMZ-TMP is popular because it is effective against a broad range of different bacteria, is available in an oral and intravenous (IV) form, is relatively inexpensive, and has a low incidence of side effects. Sulfadiazine and sulfamethoxazole are the primary sulfa drugs used in combination with trimethoprim. These antibiotics are manufactured as combination drugs because they are more effective and have fewer side effects when they are used together. Both drugs block folic acid metabolism by bacteria, but via different mechanisms. Either drug alone inhibits but does not kill susceptible bacteria. The combination, however, is bactericidal and kills susceptible bacteria.

Side Effects, Precautions, and Overdose

• Diarrhea is the most common side effect associated with oral SMZ-TMP.

• Intravenous SMZ-TMP has been associated with itching after injection and rare allergic reactions. However, some veterinarians report rare fatalities immediately after intravenous SMZ-TMP injections. Because these are anecdotal reports, it is difficult to know the cause of these fatalities.

• Injection site reactions can occur if any of the drug leaks out of the vein.

• Anemia, decreased white blood cell count, and increased blood clotting time can occur, especially with long-term use of SMZ-TMP.

• SMZ-TMP should be used with caution in horses with decreased liver function and horses with blood or bone marrow disorders.

• SMZ-TMP is generally a safe drug. No specific information was noted on overdose in the horse, but in other species overdose can cause gastrointestinal distress, central nervous system signs, and bone marrow depression. One of the manufacturers states that in horses used for safety trials a five-fold overdose caused no clinical signs.

Drug Interactions

• SMZ-TMP can increase clotting time in patients on oral antico-agulants such as warfarin.

• Antacids can decrease the absorption of SMZ-TMP. Ideally, dosing of these medications should be separated by two hours.

Special Considerations

• The label instructions on the veterinary product recommend once a day administration, but most veterinarians recommend using oral SMZ-TMP twice a day. Some use the trimethoprim sulfamethoxazole combination up to three times a day.

• Some veterinarians supplement horses on long-term SMZ-TMP with folic acid because they are concerned that folic acid metabolism in the treated animals might be impaired. This is not a concern in short-term use because the dose needed to inhibit folic acid metabolism in horses is much higher than that used to treat infections.

• SMZ-TMP is frequently used in combination with pyrimethamine in the treatment of equine protozoal myeloencephalitis. (See Pyrimethamine.)

• Trimethoprim sulfadiazine is FDA approved in the horse. Trimethoprim sulfamethoxazole is not FDA approved in the horse, but it is commonly used and an accepted practice. Both are pre-scription drugs. U.S. federal law restricts these drugs to use by or on the lawful written or oral order of a licensed veterinarian within the context of a valid veterinarian-client-patient relationship.

Special Populations

Breeding Animals

Safety of SMZ-TMP in the pregnant animal has not been clearly established. Some studies in laboratory animals have shown increased fetal losses, and one study in rats showed increased birth defects. On the other hand, many veterinarians use SMZ-TMP in pregnant mares without noticeable difficulty. SMZ-TMP crosses the placenta and is found in the milk of lactating animals. It is some-times prescribed to treat placentitis in the mare. As with most drugs, SMZ-TMP should only be used in pregnant mares when the benefits outweigh the risks. Limited work in stallions has shown no detri-mental effect on semen quality.

Foals

SMZ-TMP is frequently used in foals. Many veterinarians recom-mend that foals on SMZ-TMP be given anti-ulcer medications such as sucralfate, omeprazole, or H_2 antagonists.

Ponies

Pony breeds do not appear to differ from horses in their response to SMZ-TMP.

Geriatrics

SMZ-TMP is commonly used and appears to be safe in older hors-es with normal liver function.

Competition Horses

SMZ-TMP is not permitted in drug-free competitions, but many regulatory groups do not prohibit antibiotics or have established a permissible blood level. The drugs are not restricted by USEF for horses showing under the therapeutic substance rules. It is important to check with the individual regulatory agency.

Dose and Route of Administration

Oral: 7 to 14 mg/lb, twice a day

Injectable: 7 mg/lb, IV, twice a day. The manufacturer's recommended dose is 2 ml/100 lb, IV, one time a day, or divided into twice a day.

Dose Form:

480 mg oral tablets containing 80 mg trimethoprim and 400 mg of sulfa

960 mg oral tablets containing 160 mg trimethoprim and 800 mg sulfa

48% intravenous solution

AT A GLANCE:

XYLAZINE

GENERIC NAME
Xylazine hydrochloride

COMMON BRAND NAME
Rompun, Anased,
Sedazine, and generics

DRUG TYPE
Sedative/analgesic

INDICATIONS
Tranquilization and
pain relief

Basic Information

Xylazine is a short-acting tranquilizer or sedative that also provides significant pain relief, especially for abdominal pain. It also acts indirectly as a muscle relaxant through its effects on the central nervous system. Xylazine has a similar mechanism of action as detomidine although it is less powerful and shorter acting than detomidine.

Xylazine is a commonly used drug for short-term sedation and treatment and management of colic. The level of abdominal pain relief provided by xylazine is superior to that of many narcotics. Colic cases that are too painful to be managed by this drug are more likely to require surgery.

Xylazine is sometimes used in combination with butorphanol and other drugs for chemical restraint for many veterinary procedures or as a preoperative drug.

Xylazine is given by injection in the muscle (IM) or in the vein (IV).

Side Effects, Precautions, and Overdose

• Xylazine initially slows the heart rate and can change the heart rhythm in some horses (dropped beats).

• Horses drop their heads and appear very sedate. Moderate loss of coordination and sweating are common.

• With any form of sedation, horses can react suddenly and unexpectedly. Always work carefully around a sedated horse no matter how "asleep" it appears. Xylazine in particular has the reputation that horses may kick or react suddenly while sedated with this drug.

• Although xylazine provides some pain relief, it does not completely block pain. Horses can and will respond to painful stimulation.

• It is important to keep accurate records of xylazine and other medications used to treat a horse with colic, particularly if the animal is referred to an equine hospital for intensive care or surgery.

• Xylazine should not be used in horses with abnormal heart rhythms or heart disease. It should be used with "extreme caution" in horses with other major health problems, including shock, severe respiratory disease, and severe liver and kidney problems.

• Xylazine reduces the body's ability to regulate its temperature.

• Xylazine is a very safe drug and is tolerated at up to 10 times the recommended dose. Overdose causes heart arrhythmias, low blood pressure, and respiratory and central nervous system depression.

• Yohimbine is a drug that can be used to reverse some of the effects of xylazine.

Drug Interactions

• Xylazine has additive effects when combined with other tranquilizers and general anesthetic drugs. Although these combinations are frequently used in veterinary practice, only veterinarians experienced with the use of these drugs should do so.

Special Considerations

• Xylazine causes a drop in blood pressure but to a lesser degree than acepromazine.

• Xylazine will reliably cause a horse to drop its head when sedated. The level of sedation may vary, depending on the dose. The effect is less predictable if the horse is excited or stimulated before the drug takes full effect.

• When sedating a horse using xylazine, it is important to wait until the drug has taken effect before beginning any procedure. Sedation occurs three to five minutes after IV injection and 10 to 15 minutes after IM injection.

• Xylazine is FDA approved in the horse, and it is a prescription drug. U.S. federal law restricts this drug to use by or on the lawful written or oral order of a licensed veterinarian within the context of a valid veterinarian-client-patient relationship.

Special Populations

Breeding Animals

No information was found regarding safety during pregnancy or lactation. Clinical use of xylazine in pregnant mares has not shown detrimental effects to the mare or fetus. It is not known if xylazine is present in milk. Although stallions may relax and drop their penises when treated with xylazine, there are no reports of penile paralysis such as those with acepromazine.

Foals

Because xylazine can cause a low heart rate and slow breathing, it should be used with caution in sick foals and very young foals. Additionally, xylazine can affect an animal's ability to regulate its temperature. When xylazine is used in very young foals, the foal should remain in a temperature-controlled area until it has fully recovered. When xylazine is used in foals, it is generally used at a lower dose.

Ponies

Pony breeds do not appear to differ from horses in their response to xylazine.

Geriatrics

Xylazine should be used with caution in older animals. When xylazine is used in older horses, it is generally used at a lower dose. Reversal with yohimbine should be considered to minimize side effects.

Draft Horses

Draft horse breeds are particularly sensitive to most sedatives.

When xylazine is used in draft horse breeds, it is generally used at a lower dose.

Competition Horses

Xylazine is a prohibited substance in most sanctioned competitions. It is a prohibited class A medication under the new FEI drug rules. It may be detected for up to 72 hours. Detection may be affected by the number of doses and the sensitivity of the test. USEF has provisions in its rules for the therapeutic use of prohibited substances. It is important to check with the individual regulatory group.

Dose and Route of Administration

Injectable: 0.1 to 0.5 mg/lb, IV or IM
Dose Form: 100 mg/ml, injectable

Antibiotics Commonly Used in the Horse

Antibiotic	Administration	Commonly used for
Amikacin	Injectable IV, IM	Usually combined with other antibiotics such as penicillins. Used to treat severe mixed bacterial infections.
Ampicillin	Injectable IV, IM	Used alone for susceptible infections such as some respiratory disease. Combined with other antibiotics for severe mixed bacterial infections.
Azithromycin	Oral	*Rhodococcus* infection in foals. Combined with rifampin
Ceftiofur	Injectable IV, IM	Broad spectrum antibiotic for mixed bacterial infections including some respiratory disease. Sometimes combined with other antibiotics to broaden coverage for more severe infections.
Clarithromycin	Oral	*Rhodococcus* infection in foals. Combined with rifampin.
Chloramphenicol	Oral	Used to treat severe mixed bacterial infections. Important human health precautions.
Doxycycline	Oral	Used for mixed bacterial infections, Potomac Horse Fever, other *Ehrlichia* infections, and Lyme disease.
Enrofloxacin	Injectable:IV Oral	Broad spectrum antibiotic used for severe mixed bacterial infections. Frequently used for long-term antibiotic coverage.
Erythromycin	Oral	*Rhodococcus* infection in foals. Combined with rifampin.
Gentamicin	Injectable IV, IM	Usually combined with other antibiotics such as penicillins. Used to treat mixed bacterial infections, such as wounds, pneumonia, post surgical infections.
Metronidazole	Oral	Infections caused by anaerobic bacteria. Usually combined with other antibiotics for mixed bacterial infections.
Oxytetracycline	Injectable IV only	Used for mixed bacterial infections including respiratory disease. Drug of choice for Potomac Horse Fever and other *Ehrlichia* infections.
Penicillin G Potassium	Injectable IV only	Usually combined with other antibiotics to treat severe mixed bacterial infections. Used for some anaerobic infections, including *Clostridia*.
Procaine Penicillin	Injectable IM only	Commonly used for many minor infections including respiratory disease and wounds. Used for some anaerobic infections including *Clostridia*.
Rifampin	Oral	Used with another antibioitic, usually erythromycin, to treat *Rhodococcus* infections in foals. Not used without another antibiotic.
Ticarcillin	Injectable IV, IM	Combined with other antibiotics for severe mixed bacterial infections. Used in uterine infusions and in semen extenders.
Trimethoprim sulfa	Oral Injectable IV	Commonly used for many minor infections because of broad spectrum and ease of use.

Nonsteroidal Anti-Inflammatory Drugs Commonly Used in the Horse

NSAID	Administration	Commonly used for	Onset of Action
Aspirin	Oral	Occasionally used for pain management but more commonly used for prevention of blood clots.	Within hours
Diclofenac Sodium	Topical	Osteoarthritis and soft tissue	Within hours
Flunixin Meglumine	Oral Injectable IV or IM	Abdominal pain, fever reduction, prevention of endotoxemia, inflammation of the eye. Less commonly used for musculoskeletal pain.	Within an hour; speed of onset varies with route of administration
Ketoprofen	Injectable	Musculoskeletal pain, fever reduction, prevention of endotoxemia, abdominal pain.	Within an hour
Meclofenamic Acid	Oral	Musculoskeletal pain	Full response: 2 to 3 days
Naproxen	Oral	Musculoskeletal pain	Full response: 5 to 7 days
Phenylbutazone	Oral Injectable IV only	Musculoskeletal pain, fever reduction, general anti-inflammatory, not commonly used for colic.	Within an hour; speed of onset varies with route of administration

Index to Generic and Brand Name Drugs

Aceproject..................38

Acepromazine......38-41, 95, 97, 135, 182, 185, 189, 199, 203, 209, 212-213, 219, 223, 230-231

Acetylsalicylic acid ...56

Adequan 188

Albuterol 42-45

Altrenogest.......195-197, 200

Ambi-Pen.................176

Amiglyde...................46

Amikacin....46-47, 49, 116

Aminoglycosides...........
.:...............46-49, 74, 113

Ampicillin....176, 178, 180

Amp-Equine...........176

Anabolic steroids...........
......................50-52, 200

Anased...................229

Antihistamines....53-55, 61, 68, 134-135

Arquel 148

Aspirin 56-59, 65-66, 120, 141, 148-149, 162

Atropine 60-63, 104

Atarax 134

Azithromycin...144-147

Azium.......................83

Banamine................115

Baytril.....................112

Benzathine penicillin ...
.................176, 178-180

Betamethasone...83, 88

Betasone.............83, 88

Biaxin......................144

BismuKote 64

BismuPaste 64

Bismuth subsalicylate ...
...............................64-66

Boldenone...........50-52

Buscopan................158

Butatabs 184

Butorphanol ...67-69, 95, 211, 229

Carafate 215

Ceftiofur 70-72

Chloramphenicol.....71, 73-75, 113, 145, 209, 212

Chorulon 127

Cimetidine 58, 76-79, 101, 117, 142, 150, 156, 163, 169, 186, 215, 219

Citation....................115

Clarithromycin...144-147

Clenbuterol 42-43, 80-82

Combicillin.............176

Corrective Mixture ...64

Corticosteroids ..42, 53, 57, 77, 80, 83-88, 100, 104, 116, 120, 132, 134, 141, 149, 152, 162, 166, 170, 185, 209, 216, 222-224

Crysticillin 176

Cyproheptadine ...89-91, 182

Daraprim.................202

Depo-Medrol.............83

Deslorelin.....92-94, 128

Detomidine ...67, 95-98, 211-212, 229

Dexamethasone 83, 87-88, 167, 222, 224

Diclofenac Sodium 99-102

Dimethyl sulfoxide (DMSO).............103-106

Dinoprost 198

Dioctyl sodium sulfosuccinate (DSS).... 107-108

Dioctynate 107

Di-Trim 225

Dolorex 67

Domoso 103

Domperidone ...109-111, 174

Dormosedan.............95

Doxycycline.............65, 218-221

Durapen..................176

E-Mycin..................144

Enrofloxacin....112-114

Equidone 109

Equileve..................115

Equiphen................184

Equipoise.................50

Ery-Tab 144

Erythromycin...144-147, 178, 208-210

Flagyl 155

Flexagen 103

Flucort 83

Flumethasone 83, 88

Flunixin meglumine..... ....99, 115-118

Fulvicin...................123

Furoject 119

Furosemide ...47, 57, 85, 119-122, 162

GastroGard 169

Gentamicin ...46-47, 49, 116, 145

Gentaved..................46

Gentocin 46

Griseofulvin 123-126, 167

Histamine H2 antagonists................65

Human chorionic gonadotropin 92, 127-129

Hyaluronic acid (HA) 130-133

Hydroxyzine 134-136

Hyalovet 130

Hycoat 130

Hylartin 130

Hyvisc 130

In-Synch 198

Isoflupredone acetate ... .83, 88

Isoxsuprine hydrochloride....137-139

Ketofen 140

Ketoprofen ...99, 140-143

LA200.....................218

Lasix........................119

Legend 130

Liquamycin 218

Lutalyse 198

Macrolide antibiotics.... 144-147

Marquis 9, 192

Meclofenamic acid 148-151, 161

Meflosyl solution 115

Methocarbamol 152-154

Methylprednisolone acetate 83, 88

Metronidazole..........77, 155-157

MSM ...103, 105-106, 190

Naprosyn 161

Naproxen 161-164

Naquasone 222

Navigator.................165

Naxcel 70

N-Butylscopolammonium Bromide 158-160

Nitazoxanide...165-168, 203

Omeprazole.......58, 65, 76-77, 101, 117, 142, 145, 150, 163, 169-172, 186, 215, 227

Ovuplant...........92, 128

Oxoject.....................173

Oxytetracycline ...218-221

Oxytocin....81, 173-175, 199

Penicillin 176-180

Pen-G 176

PeptoBismol..............64

Periactin 89

Pergolide 90, 181-183

Permax.....................181

Pfi-Pen G 176

Phenylbutazone...57, 99, 116-117, 141, 184-187

Phenylzone 184

Pitocin.....................173

Polysulfated Glycosaminoglycan....... ....188, 190-191

Ponazuril 9, 192-194, 203

Potassium Penicillin 176

Predef 2X.................83

Prednisone 195-197

Procaine Penicillin........ ....176-178, 180

Progesterone   109, 195-198, 200

Promace....................38

Promazine Granules...38

Promazine hydrochloride............38

Prostaglandin.....81, 84, 99, 189-190, 198-201

ProstaMate 198

Protostat 155

Proventil 42

Pyrilaject...................53

Pyrilamine..........53-55

Pyrimethamine 193, 202-204, 226

Ranitidine ...76-79, 169, 215, 219

Rebalance................202

Re-Covr....................53

Regu-Mate 195-196

Reserpine 205-207

Rifadin....................208

Rifampin 208-210

Rimactane 208

Robaxin 152

Robimycin..............144

Rompun...................229

Romifidine 211-214

SMZ-TMP 202-203, 225-227

Sedazine 229

Sedivet 211

Solu-Delta-Cortef......83

Stanozolol 50-52

Sucralfate ...58, 65, 76-77, 101, 113, 117, 142, 150, 163, 169, 186, 215-217, 227

Sulfadiazine 202, 225-226

Surpass 99

Tagamet 76

Terramycin 218

Tetracycline antibiotics 65, 218-221

Ticarcillin 176-180

Ticar 176

Ticillin 176

Torbugesic 67

Triamcinolone.....83, 88

Tribrissen.................225

Trichlormethiazide 222-224

Trimethoprim sulfa ...96, 120, 209, 212, 225-228

Tripelennamine ...53-55

UlcerGard...............169

Ventipulmin 80

Ventolin 42

Vetalog 83

Vibramycin..............218

Vistaril 134

Vita Flex MSM........103

Winstrol 50

Xylazine.............67, 95, 211-212, 229-232

Zantac 76

Zithromax 144

References

Much of the information in this book may be found in the following reference texts. I have included a short comment after each reference to guide the reader seeking additional information.

American Association of Equine Practitioners Annual Convention Proceedings, Lexington, KY.: AAEP, 1995-2005.

American Association of Equine Practitioners Resource Library, Guidelines to Drug Detection Times. Volumes 1 and 2. Lexington, KY: AAEP, 1999 and 2000.
   The AAEP publications are always a good source of up-to-date scientific and clinical information. Written for veterinarians.

Bertone JJ, Horspool LJI, edits. *Equine Clinical Pharmacology*. Philadelphia: W.B. Saunders, 2004.
   This is an excellent recent text.

Colahan PT, Mayhew IG, Merritt AM, Moore JN, edits. *Equine Medicine and Surgery*. 5th edition. St. Louis, MO: Mosby, 1999.
   Everything you ever wanted to know if you were an equine veterinarian. Written for veterinarians.

Hinchcliffe KW, Sams RA, edits. *Veterinary Clinics of North America: Equine Practice: Drug Use in Performance Horses*: Volume 9, No. 3. Philadelphia: W.B. Saunders, December 1993.
   Veterinary Clinics *is a series of short specialty books with articles written by veterinary experts on a variety of topics. Written for veterinarians.*

Kellon EM. *Equine Drugs and Vaccines*. Ossining, N.Y.: Breakthrough Publications, 1995.
   A larger book covering drugs, vaccines, and diseases of the horse. Dr. Thomas Tobin wrote some of the chapters and consulted on this book. There is an emphasis on racing. Written for lay persons.

McKinnon AO, Voss JL, edits. *Equine Reproduction*. Philadelphia: Lea and Febiger, 1993.
A reference text on equine reproduction written by reproductive specialists and veterinarians. Written for veterinarians.

Physician's Desk Reference (PDR). 55th edition. Montvale, N.J.: Medical Economics, 2001.
The PDR gives the package inserts for human drugs.

Plumb DC. *Veterinary Drug Handbook*. 5th edition. Ames, IA.: Iowa State University Press, 2005.
Plumb is a classic reference text that lists hundreds of drugs that are used in veterinary medicine. Written for veterinarians.

Ramey DW. *Concise Guide to Medications and Supplements for the Horse*. New York: Howell Book House, 1996.
One of the "Concise Guide" *series. This book has brief descriptions of many prescription drugs, over-the-counter drugs, and supplements. Written for lay persons.*

Robinson NE, edit. *Current Therapy in Equine Medicine*. Volumes 3 and 4. Philadelphia: W.B. Saunders, 1992, 1997, 2002.
This is a great series that contains articles on medical problems of the horse written by veterinary experts. Written for veterinarians.

Tobin T. *Drugs in Performance Horses*. Springfield, IL: Charles C. Thomas, 1981.
A very clear and understandable book on drugs and their use and abuse in performance horses. Unfortunately, it is getting a little old. A second edition would be great. Written for lay persons and veterinarians.

Veterinary Pharmaceuticals and Biologicals (VPB). Lenexa, KS: Veterinary Medicine Publishing Group, 2001-2002.
The VPB *gives the package inserts for veterinary drugs.*

Photo Credits

Tom Hall, 10; Anne M. Eberhardt, 27; Paula da Silva, 30
Photo well: Dr. Steve Berkowitz

Acknowledgments

This book is dedicated to the memory of Dr. Rachel Pemstein, a good friend and a great veterinarian. Rachel and I dreamed up this book together, and I am sorry she is not with us to see it come true.

I would like to thank the following individuals who in particular helped make this book possible:

Always first, my husband, children, and the rest of my family, who were always full of support and encouragement. Thanks to my friend Dr. Lenny Southam, who read and commented on every word along the way; this is a better book for her wisdom and humor. Also, thanks go to Sue Haldeman for her skill, insight, and encouragement.

Thanks to my friends at Petra, who gave me more good reasons to stay at my desk and write. Last, but not least, thanks to my clients/friends and their horses. They are a constant source of education, inspiration, and humor.

About the Author

Barbara D. Forney, MS, VMD, grew up in Wilmington, Delaware, in a family of chemical engineers and spent most of her youth plotting how to ride and spend more time around horses. Fortunately, Wilmington is close to Chester County, Pennsylvania, which is wonderful horse country.

After undergraduate school she worked first for Dr. Al Merritt in the Section of Medicine and then with Drs. Robert Kenney and Wendell Cooper in the Section of Reproduction at the University of Pennsylvania School of Veterinary Medicine's Large Animal Hospital at New Bolton Center. While working in the Section of 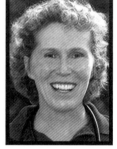 Reproduction, she received a master's degree in animal science in 1978 from the University of Delaware. She graduated from veterinary school at the University of Pennsylvania in 1982 and entered private practice in the immediate area.

The Chester County area is home to a wide variety of horses and horse sports. Forney's practice interests have been primarily medicine and reproduction, with an additional mix of sport horses. Because combined training is such a major sport in that area, she became involved in taking care of three-day-event horses, competing in lower levels events, organizing horse trials, and working as a veterinarian at major three-day and combined driving events around the country. Forney is an FEI veterinarian; a career highlight was being a part of the veterinary team at the Atlanta Olympic Games in 1996.

In 1999 Forney spent a year studying breeding behavior of stallions while participating in a research fellowship with the Havemeyer Foundation. She has returned to private practice and continues to consult on reproductive problems of horses. She lives with her family and pets outside of Unionville, Pennsylvania, where they breed event and pleasure horses.